THE Z FA

Current scientific research is highlighting the lack of the
mineral zinc as a crucial factor in a wide range of disorders.
Here, the authors show why zinc is so important to health,
how to find out if you are lacking in this mineral and how to
boost the crucial Z factor in your diet.

THE Z FACTOR

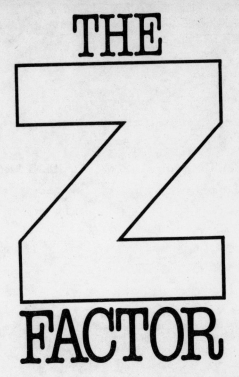

FACTOR

How Zinc is Vital to Your Health

Judy Graham and Dr Michel Odent

THORSONS PUBLISHING GROUP
Wellingborough, Northamptonshire
Rochester, Vermont

First published 1986

British Library Cataloguing in Publication Data

Graham, Judy
The Z factor: how zinc is vital to your health.
1. Zinc — Physiological effect
I. Title   II. Odent, Michel
613.2'8   QP913.Z6

ISBN 0-7225-1329-1

Printed and bound in Great Britain

Contents

Introduction

In the last few years zinc has proved to be one of the keys to good health. Before that it had been just another mystery — something we vaguely knew was needed, but without being aware precisely why. In fact, only a decade ago the true importance of zinc was largely unrealized, and if you open any biochemistry textbook published before 1970 as likely as not there'll be no mention — or hardly any mention — of zinc at all. Then, all of a sudden, there was an explosion of interest.

Zinc is essential. In fact zinc is needed for so many things that you could almost compile a dictionary of the conditions in which zinc plays a role. There are hardly any instances of the diseases common in our civilization where either a lack of zinc or an incorrect use of zinc by the body are not subjects of research studies.

Of these, perhaps the most interesting — and the one which arouses most passion — is reproduction. Zinc is involved in all aspects of it — male impotence, genital development, sterility, foetal development, difficulties in childbirth, difficulties in breastfeeding and sexual problems.

We now know that a human being absorbs about 400kg of zinc in the course of a normal lifespan and at any one time there are 2g - 3g of zinc in the body. Zinc is needed at every age and every stage of life, starting with the foetus and finishing with old age. A lack of zinc can cause retardation of foetal growth, and the process of ageing cannot be properly studied without understanding how important zinc is in metabolism.

At last, many medical disciplines are beginning to discover the enormous therapeutic uses for zinc. Mothers have known for generations that the best thing for nappy rash was zinc and castor oil cream. But it is only recently that dermatologists have known how good zinc is for acne, eczema, stretch marks and for hair and nails.

Zinc hit the headlines when psychiatrists began to use zinc supplements for anorexia nervosa. It seemed at last that there was a solution to this enigma. Less publicized, but no less important, zinc has been used in the treatment of depression, schizophrenia and autism.

When it comes to common childhood illnesses, some paediatricians are now beginning to think of zinc for things like ear, nose and throat infections, chicken pox and measles. General practitioners are also turning their thoughts to zinc. Many illnesses affecting the digestive system demand more zinc — something which no one suspected before, and it would be impossible to measure the influence zinc will have in the prevention and treatment of prostate troubles which affect so many older men. In fact, every speciality, even including intensive care, where people are fed intravenously, must now think about how much zinc their patients might need.

As will be seen later on in the book, zinc is a vital component in the immune system if such a system is to function correctly. So this makes zinc important in a great multitude of conditions where the immume system seems to have gone wrong, including allergies, auto-immune diseases, viral diseases and cancers.

Landmarks in the History of Zinc Research

How is it that in just a few years there has been a shift from indifference to passion about zinc? After all, the discoveries about zinc and what it could do were not made overnight. It has only been during the 1980s that awareness of the value of zinc really took off, biochemists revealing that zinc was everywhere, acting as an important catalyst in every metabolic process.

It will be no surprise to discover that traditional Chinese medicine knew about 'Lin-suan-hsin' centuries ago. It's what we would call zinc sulphate. The Chinese used it for prostate problems. The ancient Egyptians also knew about zinc and how useful it could be for health. Then there was a very long gap in the history of zinc, right up to this century. In the 1950s zinc was suddenly in the limelight for its starring role in a pig disease called keratose. It was found that this common skin disease among pigs could be successfully treated with zinc, which only goes to show how far ahead veterinary medicine was compared with human medicine. These pigs gave a Virginian farmer an idea: the farmer's son had bad acne, and he wondered whether the treatment that had worked so well on the pigs might have a similar success on his son. The farmer's hunch proved correct — the zinc which had cured the skin disease in the pigs worked the same way on his son's acne. And that, believe it or not, was how zinc first came to be used in the treatment of acne.

At the end of the 1960s it was discovered that a lack of zinc could actually cause a very severe condition — a hereditary skin disease called acrodermatitis enteropathica.

The Wider Issues Concerning Zinc

This book is about zinc and health. But it would be a mistake to describe it as a book which is just about a new topic in nutrition. It goes far beyond that. It raises the issue of what it is in our society which makes modern man need more zinc than he ever used to. Man's increased need for zinc today calls into question many aspects of modern-day life, including orthodox medicine, obstetrics, neonatology and the pollution of our world.

Zinc can never be considered on its own. Other minerals can make you need more of it — especially copper. This is not just in foods, but in the whole environment. Once you know this, you can see how zinc suddenly becomes an issue in, for example, methods of contraception and even domestic plumbing. Both the pill and the copper coil exaggerate the effects of any lack of zinc, and copper pipes in the plumbing have a similar effect.

When you discover just how much zinc is needed by modern man, you are struck by the enormous implications of this — going far beyond the usual spheres of biologists, nutritionists and doctors.

Modern farming and food processing techniques are also probably making you need more zinc than ever before. Zinc is being robbed from soils because of the widespread use of phosphate fertilizers, and zinc is lost in certain refining processes practised by the food industry.

There are many other reasons too why people living in the western world today may be short of zinc, and these are discussed in this book. It is something of an ironic situation. There can be no previous time in history when so many foods were available, many of them rich in zinc, yet the stark truth is that zinc deficiency is widespread, and many conditions point to a lack of zinc.

Is the World Suffering from a Zinc Deficiency?

Doctors who have made nutritional medicine their speciality are horrified by the low levels of zinc in western populations. Dr Carl Pfeiffer states: 'Under the best of circumstances, the level of zinc in any modern diet may be minimal, contaminated, or downright missing. Hence the need for zinc supplements.'

The Recommended Daily Allowances (RDAs), in those countries which have set them, are considered woefully inadequate, and it seems that zinc is one of the major nutrient deficiencies in both industrialized nations and in the Third World, although for different reasons.

1
Zinc and Your Health

How Zinc Works in the Body

Zinc has many different functions in the body. When you see how varied these are, you can understand why a zinc deficiency can have such widespread results, and why it can be so serious. Zinc is essential for the production of proteins and the synthesis of DNA — the basis of the genetic code. Zinc is essential for the formation of nucleic acid which controls protein formation within the cells. This means that zinc has an important role in regulating the controlling influence of genes on the synthesis of new tissues in the body, and that zinc is crucial in the process of cell division and growth.

Zinc forms part of the composition of at least 160 different enzymes. Indeed, zinc is the most widely used mineral in enzymes. These enzymes are involved in digestion, metabolism and tissue respiration. It is known that enzymes containing zinc are needed by the body for the production and efficiency of both DNA and RNA (ribonucleic acid). One of these metallo-enzymes is called carbonic anhydrase. This removes carbon dioxide, as bicarbonate, from tissues. It also assists the kidneys in producing the ammonium ion for excretion, and it produces gastric hydrochloric acid.

Zinc also takes a leading role in the processes which ensure normal absorption and function of vitamins, especially the B group, and zinc is a co-factor in the production of collagen. It is collagen which helps keep tissues rigid.

A Healthy Immune System

Zinc is needed in the metabolism of essential fatty acids from which prostaglandins are produced. This means that the immune system cannot work properly without zinc. Because zinc's role in the synthesis of prostaglandins is so vital, and because this comes up again throughout this book, it is worth going into some detail about this particular metabolic process.

Prostaglandins are cell regulators which work a bit like local hormones. They are very short-lived and work on a second-by-second basis regulating each and every cell in every tissue and every organ of your body.

The prostaglandins are grouped into series 1, 2 and 3. We are mostly concerned with prostaglandins series 1, as they have a particularly important role to play in the health of the immune system. PG 1 also have an action on the small blood vessels, helping them to dilate and so reducing blood-pressure. They also stop the platelets in the blood from bunching up together, and so prevent blood clots from forming. PG 1 also inhibit the synthesis of cholesterol, and reduce inflammation. Zinc has an important role to play in the synthesis of PG 1.

The prostaglandins series 2 are involved in inflammatory processes. There is a sort of see-saw, or feedback mechanism, between PG 1 and PG 2. When the level of PG 1 goes up, the level of PG 2 goes down, and vice versa. Ideally, there should be a balance between these two series of prostaglandins, and also between different prostaglandins in the same series. Zinc plays an important role in maintaining this balance.

The Role of Zinc in the Production of Prostaglandins

Zinc is a catalyst which is needed in the metabolism of linoleic acid on its path towards prostaglandins 1 (linoleic acid must be in the 'cis' form — see page 36.) Zinc plays its part at the first stage of this metabolic process, when linoleic acid is converted into gammalinolenic acid; and it also works at the next stage, when gammalinolenic acid is converted to the precursor of prostaglandins 1.

Gammalinolenic acid (GLA) is an almost direct precursor of PG 1. But that doesn't mean it always ends up as PG 1. It can still take a detour and end up as PG 2 instead. This is where zinc comes in — it helps maintain a balance between the different series of prostaglandins, as well as playing an essential role in all the chemical reactions which lead to PG 1.

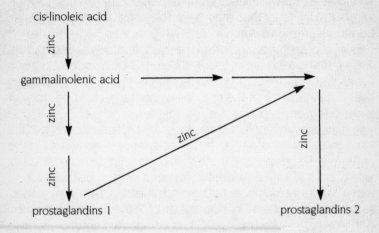

Figure 1. The role of zinc in the production of prostaglandins

The Role of Zinc in the Immune System

So, zinc is a vital catalyst in the metabolism of essential fatty acids, from which prostaglandins 1 are produced. Apart from their many other functions in the body, prostaglandins 1 are indispensable for the good workings of the immune system. PG 1 have some similar actions to thymic hormone, and they seem to be necessary for the normal functioning of T lymphocytes.

The white cells, called lymphocytes, after having developed in the bone marrow, mature in the thymus. That's why they're called 'T' lymphocytes. These 'T' lymphocytes are the body's army, so they are essential if the immune system is to defend itself properly. Some of these T lymphocytes become T killers, which can destroy their targets; others become T helpers which can help other white cells make antibodies; and others become T suppressors which moderate the manufacture of antibodies.

The thymus is an essential organ of the immune system. It is a gland situated behind the sternum. Its size decreases after puberty, and there is hardly anything left of it in old people. There is an abundance of prostaglandins 1 in the thymus. It has been shown in laboratory tests that they have the same actions as thymic hormones in the maturation of T lymphocytes.

Zinc plays an important role in the specialization of lymphocytes, and in the balance between the different T cells. Indeed, a good balance of the different types of lymphocytes is a sign of good health. The activity of the thymic hormones is also tied up with there being enough zinc.

Something very significant was found by an Italian research team: the concentration of active thymic hormones is very weak in the plasma of old people and those with Down's Syndrome — in other words, people with a weakened immune system. But they found that adding zinc sulphate to the plasma was all that was needed to re-establish a normal concentration of active thymic hormones. Another study looked at the effects of zinc on the immune response of some patients with Down's Syndrome and the results were highly significant. Zinc has the same effect on diseases such as kidney disease, when the patient is on dialysis, and sickle cell anaemia. Babies born with sickle cell anaemia have a depressed immune system and it is difficult for them to resist infections, but zinc supplements have a spectacular effect in helping to reinforce their immune systems.

Zinc, Enzymes and Free Radicals

Within body cells, zinc is complexed with a variety of proteins, peptides and amino acids, including dozens of enzymes. The best known of these enzymes are carbonic anhydrase (see page 11), alcohol dehydrogenase, lactic dehydrogenase, pancreatic carboxypeptidase and superoxide dismutase (S.O.D.). Any changes in the enzymes complex will immediately be reflected in changes in the whole prostaglandin cascade.

It is S.O.D. which seems to be particularly important. S.O.D. is an anti-oxidant enzyme (in fact this is not a single enzyme but a group of enzymes) which has a role in combatting free radicals in the body.

It is known that in some circumstances, for example high temperatures, the molecules of unsaturated fatty acids accept oxygen atoms more easily. This is part of the oxidation process. The oxidation process chops fatty acids out of the membranes. These oxygen atoms can then detach themselves and fix onto another molecule. These unstable molecules which transport oxygen are called 'free radicals'. Free radicals can be destructive. There is a loss of integrity of the membranes. All functional controls go by the board and anarchy takes over. They are implicated in certain diseases such as cancer and arteriosclerosis. So the whole anti-oxidant system is very important. It includes minerals such as selenium, vitamins such as C and E (natural vitamin E works best) and enzymes — superoxide dismutase in particular. So, here again, zinc is involved in a vital chemical reaction in the body. However, as well as zinc, manganese, iron, and copper are also involved in the function of S.O.D.

Where Else Zinc Is Needed in the Body

Zinc is needed for the release of insulin by the pancreas, and for the release of vitamin A from its liver stores, and it has an important role to play in the metabolism of the pituitary gland, the adrenal glands, the ovaries and the testes. Zinc is vital for the production of male sperm and female ova, it is necessary for a healthy liver metabolism and it is needed by the foetus in order to grow properly.

Zinc Deficiency — The Signs and Symptoms

When you look at the things zinc does in the body, it is easy to see how some signs and symptoms can point to a lack of zinc. This is because zinc deficiency has a broad effect on all enzyme activity, as well as on the synthesis of prostaglandins.

One London biochemist who tests people for zinc deficiency says he can pick out people lacking in zinc as they walk down the street. 'They are lack-lustre in their hair and skin,' he says.

Signs of zinc deficiency include: poor skin; delayed wound healing; stretch marks — especially over the hips, thighs, abdomen, breasts and shoulders; poor hair condition, sometimes with loss of pigment and hair loss; loss of sense of taste and smell; loss of appetite; apathy and lethargy; white flecks on the nails, which are also likely to be brittle. For some reason, Sweden seems a particularly bad place for zinc deficiency. Many of the medical photos used to illustrate poor hair, poor skin and white flecks on the nails were taken in Sweden.

Other signs of a possible zinc deficiency include poor protein and carbohydrate metabolism; retarded growth; slow mental development; defects in the reproductive organs; bizarre food cravings during pregnancy (pica); and increased susceptibility to infections.

Conditions Where the Immune System Has Gone Wrong

Zinc works in a number of ways to reinforce the immune system. That is why the use of zinc is relevant to the enormous number of conditions which involve some defect in the immune system. This includes allergy problems like hayfever, asthma, eczema and urticaria (all of which are very common) and all the auto-immune diseases, where the immune system attacks its own body instead of protecting it. Any part of the body can come under attack in an auto-immune disease. It could be the pancreas, ending up as diabetes; it could be the thyroid, ending up as thyroiditis; it could be the digestive tract, ending up as stomach ulcers, or ulcerative colitis or Crohn's disease. Sometimes the attack is diffuse and ends up as systemic lupus or a rheumatic disease.

There are a large number of viral diseases and they, too, can be helped along by a weak immune system. It's a vicious circle; the virus can act as a blocking agent in the synthesis of prostaglandins, and this can itself depress the immune system. And just to make things more complicated, some auto-immune diseases might be triggered by viruses. There is a suspicion that this is the case in diabetes and multiple sclerosis, though whether they are classified as auto-immune or viral diseases makes no practical difference.

Cancer comes under the heading of a dysfunction of the immune system. So does ageing and, perhaps less obviously, some forms of sterility and some instances of miscarriage. It has been shown that women who had several miscarriages were not making certain antibodies which a woman normally has to make in order to tolerate the presence of what amounts to a foreign body — her own baby. There are now treatments where the future mother is injected with the white blood cells of her partner before conception, so she can make the necessary antibodies in advance.

Vitamin B$_6$ and Zinc

Zinc teams up with vitamin B$_6$ in the body, particularly for protein synthesis. It has been found that people who are lacking in vitamin B$_6$ cannot handle proteins properly. But once they are given an adequate amount of B$_6$ they are able to handle proteins in the normal way.

Dr Carl Pfeiffer, of the Brain Bio Center in New Jersey, has found that in many conditions, patients are deficient in both zinc and B$_6$. He calls this 'pyroluria' — they are losing zinc and B$_6$ in the urine.

Multiple sclerosis and schizophrenia are two such 'pyroluric' conditions. In Dr Pfeiffer's experience, both respond very well to B$_6$ and zinc together. With MS, Dr Pfeiffer has reported: 'No further progression of the disease — individuals are frequently stabilized.' Schizophrenia is discussed in Chapter 13. Dr Pfeiffer claims astonishing results with schizophrenic patients using zinc and B$_6$.

It seems that our needs for zinc and B$_6$ are increased in what physiologists call situations of helplessness and hopelessness, i.e.

situations in which we have no control. These are connected with a high level of the hormone cortisol (see page 39).

B_6 is such an important team-mate of zinc that it is not enough to have yourself tested for your mineral status alone. You also need to know your biochemical status at the same time in order to have the full picture.

Conditions in Which a Lack of Zinc May Be Involved

The list of conditions in which a lack of zinc has been shown to be involved, or is thought to be involved, is almost long enough to fill a medical dictionary. An A-Z of them would include the following:

Acne
Acrodermatitis Enteropathica
Alcoholism — Chronic
Anorexia Nervosa
Arteriosclerosis
Atherosclerosis
Autism
Body Odour
Boils
Cirrhosis of the Liver
Coeliac Disease
Colds
Cold Sores
Crohn's Disease
Cystic Fibrosis
Depression
Diabetes
Down's Syndrome
Dyslexia
Eczema
Foetal Abnormalities

Foetal Growth Retardation
Geophagia (clay eating)
Growth Retardation
Herpes
High Blood-Pressure
Hyperactivity in Children
Impotence
Infections — Chronic
Infertility
Intravenous Feeding
Kidney Dialysis — long term
Learning Difficulties
Leg Ulcers
Low-Birth-Weight Babies
Malnutrition (low protein/
    high carbohydrate diets)
Mouth Ulcers
Multiple Sclerosis (and
    other auto-immune
    diseases)
Muscular Tics

Nanism (Dwarfism)
Pancreatic Disease
Photophobia
Pica
Post-Natal Depression
Pregnancy
Prostate problems
Rheumatoid Arthritis and other inflammatory conditions
Rosacea
Schizophrenia
Sexual Development —
retarded growth
Sickle Cell Anaemia
Skin Complaints
Stress from Surgery or Burns
Stretch Marks
Taste — loss of
Thalassaemia
TB
Ulcerative Colitis
Whitlows
Wilson's Disease
Wound Healing — delayed

Some of these conditions are discussed in this book, although it is beyond the scope of a book this size to go into detail about each and every one of them.

Low zinc levels are also found in women who are on the contraceptive pill, and in patients on corticosteroid drugs — who either take them in high doses or over a long period of time. Also, breastfeeding mothers can be short of zinc. Smokers, and people who regularly breathe in other people's smoke (passive smokers) can be low in zinc as well.

The whole subject of how much zinc you need and why some people need more zinc than others is discussed fully in Chapter 3.

2
Zinc and a New Kind of Medicine

An increased need for zinc is one of the common ties between all the different diseases of civilization. Zinc's importance in the immune system is well known and based on hard facts, but it is a very rare doctor who first checks that the patient is eating a diet which contains an optimum amount of the nutrients for the synthesis of prostaglandins and the working of the thymus. Instead of prescribing immuno-suppressive drugs straightaway, a doctor might ask questions such as these:

*   Is the patient getting enough of the raw materials — the essential fatty acids — to be able to make prostaglandins 1?
*   Is the patient getting enough of the essential catalysts, especially zinc?
*   Is the patient getting enough of the co-factors of zinc, especially vitamin B_6 and vitamin C, magnesium, the other B vitamins and selenium?
*   Might the patient's body contain too much of the minerals which increase the need for zinc, such as cadmium, copper and lead?
*   Is the patient reducing his or her intake of processed fats, sugar and alcohol?
*   Is the patient taking in a good balance of all the vitamins and minerals?

Doctors who do approach things in this way are very much in the minority, although their numbers are growing. This approach aims to boost the immune system. It is very different from that of orthodox medicine which normally resorts to drugs which dampen down the immune system and which tackle only the symptoms.

'Nouvelle Medicine'

We have coined the name 'Nouvelle Medicine'. A medicine which tries first of all to understand basic human needs, and to satisfy them.

'Nouvelle Medicine' is not concerned with pigeon-holing all the various conditions. Indeed, it would prefer that the man-made barriers which section off one disease from another into different specialities were broken down. In conventional medical research, some scientists research cancer; others research rheumatism; others research viral diseases; others research allergies; others research multiple sclerosis, and so on. But the different 'diseases of civilization' seem more and more to be just different masks disguising the same disease. Whether it comes out as cancer, or an auto-immune disease, or something else, may depend on a person's genetic constitution and the age at which they had to face difficult situations.

Research in 'Nouvelle Medicine' is much more interested in the *genesis* of good health, and not on the prevention and treatment of a particular disease. It is also interested in simple diagnostic procedures and simple practical measures. Anyone faced with a disease which affects the immune system, a chronic disease which threatens to last a lifetime, will have to decide what course of action to take.

The guidelines of 'Nouvelle Medicine' are very different from the orthodox approach:

(i)   Think carefully before taking aggressive drugs. Such drugs have only short-term effects on the symptoms, but the long term should also be considered. From the outset, regard corti-costeroids with suspicion. (Be careful! There are several different types with a variety of different names.) Treat in the same way all the other drugs which depress the immune system (especially cyclosporin). The frightening number of prescriptions for these drugs is not based on any long-term study.

(ii)   Immediately increase your intake of zinc, vitamin C, vitamin B_6, and unsaturated fatty acids. Instil this dietary habit into yourself and keep it up for the rest of your life, day in, day out.

(iii) Try to organize your lifestyle so that it is less stressful. In this way you will secrete less cortisol. It will mean doing your best to change your attitude towards life. Don't be scared of taking your destiny into your own hands, and making decisions about your life. Avoid situations of dependency and submission. Avoid mixing with pessimists.

Conventional medicine is a long way off from this. If you mention to a conventional doctor that you are following the above regime, and taking zinc and other vitamins and minerals every day, you are likely to be met with a polite smile and be told that it would be necessary to do long-term double blind controlled trials to evaluate such a regime.

It seems that conventional medicine is reluctant to accept ideas from lay people, and it would be very interesting to study the acceptability of a particular therapy for a particular disease depending on where the idea to use it first came from. For instance, why are nearly all babies considered to be lacking in vitamin K at birth, when no study has ever proved the usefulness of a routine injection? And why are so many newborn babies exposed to light which prevents them from turning yellow when no study has ever proved that the advantages of this outweigh the disadvantages?

However, there are many therapists taking the 'Nouvelle Medicine' approach who are sure they have helped ill people by using zinc and its co-factors. This applies to a wide range of illnesses, including auto-immune diseases, allergic diseases, viral diseases and cancer.

Some Simple Diagnostic Procedures

Part of 'Nouvelle Medicine' is the use of simple diagnostic

procedures — tests that can be used by a doctor either at his surgery or at the patient's home. For zinc deficiency there are two very simple diagnostic tests. One is the detection of white spots on the nails, introduced by Dr Carl Pfeiffer, a founder of the Brain Bio Center in Princeton, New Jersey. And the other is the 'Taste Test' advocated by Professor Derek Bryce-Smith of Reading University, and now on sale through some companies for home use. These diagnostic tests are explained in detail on pages 44 and 45.

3
Where Does Zinc Come From?

The first thing to say is that the amount of zinc in a particular food is not as important as how well it can be used by the body — its bio-availability. Minerals in general are not nearly so well absorbed as other nutrients. Fats, carbohydrates, proteins and vitamins usually have 100% absorption, whereas most minerals only have 10-15% absorption.

Zinc and Infant Feeding

For a baby, the main source of zinc is its mother's milk. Human breast milk contains about 0.3mg of zinc per dl, or 0.4mg for 100kg cal, although there is quite a wide variation between one mother and another. There is a lot of zinc in colostrum, the stuff which precedes the milk.

Cow's milk has more zinc in it. But when you compare human breast milk with cow's milk for the bio-availability of its content, breast milk comes out on top — about 60% compared with only 30% - 40% for cow's milk.

There are several reasons why the zinc in breast milk is more bio-available. First, the zinc in breast milk binds itself to a substance, called a ligand, of low molecular weight which is specific to human milk. Second, cow's milk contains much more phosphate. The zinc combines with the phosphate and so is less available. In any case, a breastfed baby probably needs less zinc than a bottlefed baby.

Human breast milk contains some very special essential fatty acids, gammalinolenic acid in particular (GLA). Zinc acts as a catalyst in the metabolism of essential fatty acids. Indeed, this is one of the most important functions of zinc. So a breastfed baby is getting both GLA and zinc from its mother's milk. But what about the bottlefed baby?

Of course, the manufacturers of formula milk are well aware of a baby's needs, including its needs for zinc. The Committee on Nutrition of the American Academy of Pediatrics recommends that artificial milks contain a minimum of 0.5mg of zinc per 100kg cal, and the manufacturers abide by these recommendations. There is also a formula feed designed especially for premature babies ('Similac' Special Care) which contains 1.2mg of zinc per dl. The higher zinc content is because premature babies were thought to have a zinc deficiency because the transfer of zinc from mother to baby is known to take place mostly in the last ten weeks of pregnancy. But, in fact, the real cause of these apparent deficiencies might be too much iron in the formula. Iron makes the absorption of zinc more difficult. With premature babies, when the iron/zinc ratio goes above 3:1 what might be called for are zinc supplements.

Balance Between Minerals

This raises the important issue of balance. If zinc is going to work properly, there has to be a balance between the various minerals ingested. What seems on the face of it to be a zinc deficiency may in fact be the result of ingesting too much of another mineral or minerals, such as iron.

This question of balance between the minerals starts during infancy, the period when the baby is dependent on its mother. The baby's diet at this time plays a key role in its future dietary adaptation. Human breast milk contains only 0.05mg per dl of iron. Artificial milks usually contain more than this, sometimes as much as twenty times more. This is surely too much. Breast milk contains the perfect balance of zinc and iron (as well as all the other nutrients).

Unfortunately, in western society, babies are not often breastfed for very long, so few babies start out with an ideal nutritional balance.

It is worth making the point that there are no reported examples of negative effects of an excess of zinc during infancy.

The Food Sources of Zinc

Zinc can be found almost everywhere; in the soil, in the sea, in animals, in plants.

Some of the foods with most zinc are:

	mg zinc per 100g
Oysters	45-70
Liver	7.8
Brewer's yeast	7.8
Shrimps	5.3
Crab	5.0
Beef	4.3
Cheese	4.0
Sardines	3.0
Canned ham	2.3
Wholemeal bread	2.0

Most zinc is found in the organ meats of animals, such as liver, brain and kidneys. The best sources of zinc are certainly from animals and seafood.

Dairy products are also important sources of zinc. Cheese has the most, depending on the type:

	mg zinc per 100g
Cheddar cheese	4
Edam	4
Camembert	3.0
White cheese	0.47
Egg	1.8
Butter	0.15

In the UK, at least 75% of dietary zinc comes from meat, fish, eggs and dairy products.

Lower down the list in the zinc league table are vegetables, grains and pulses. For example, peas have 0.7mg; carrots 0.4mg; rice 0.35mg; potatoes 0.29mg; green beans 0.21mg; and tomatoes 0.2mg per 100g. When foods are commercially frozen (e.g. peas, broccoli, spinach) a large percentage of the zinc is lost.

Humans do not keep reserves of zinc, so every day you really have to eat some foods which contain zinc. From the above lists it's obvious that if you eat foods of animal origin you'll be getting much more zinc than somebody who eats no meat or fish. Vegans, who eat no foods of animal origin, will be getting the least zinc from their diet.

As well as having the most zinc, foods of animal origin have zinc in its most bio-available form. The zinc in these foods is in a form which makes it easily and efficiently used because animal proteins are rich in cysteine, an amino acid which helps the zinc to be absorbed.

What If You're Vegetarian?

Recently, healthy eating has become synonymous with being vegetarian. But there is a catch. Foods from plant sources have less zinc. Not only that, but the zinc in these foods is often not bio-available except in tiny amounts. Why is this?

Phytic Acid

First, most vegetables — cereals in particular — contain phytic acid. Phytic acid (or inositol hexaphosphate to give it its proper name) has the property of combining with certain metals — zinc in particular — in such a way that the phytates cannot be absorbed by the digestive tract. When the ratio between phytic acid and zinc goes above 15:1 the bio-availability of zinc is virtually zero.

Some of the most popular cereal products have the following phytic acid/zinc ratios.

Wholemeal flour	35:1
Wholemeal bread	33:1
Oats	27:1
Cornflakes	21:1
White bread	15:1
White flour	13:1

Meat products using soya flour and other cereals have very high phytic acid/zinc ratios, often over 35:1. The hamburger is typical of this group.

When bread is baked traditionally, it is a good source of zinc. At least 50% of the phytic acid is destroyed, thanks to the enzyme phytase which is found in wheat and yeast. And the high temperature of the oven completes the destruction of phytic acid. But, by contrast, modern techniques of bread manufacture destroy only a small part of the phytic acid.

On the face of it, all this makes gloomy reading for vegetarians and those who subsist on hamburgers. But there seems to be a real difference between people who have always been vegetarian, and people who switched to being vegetarian once they were adults. It seems that it all depends on whether you can use the enzyme phytase or not. It seems that people who have grown up on vegetarian diets are able to use phytase, which liberates zinc from the phytic acid mineral complex, whereas people who have switched to vegetarianism do not have this particular enzyme at their disposal.

People who have always been vegetarian will need less zinc because they have the active phytase enzyme. However, adults who suddenly become vegetarians, without any transition from meat-eating, will not have developed phytase; so they will need more zinc.

Fibre

The fibre in vegetables is another reason why there is poor bio-availability of zinc in vegetarian diets. Fibre is not digested in the intestine, whether it's hard fibre from grains or soft fibre from fruits and vegetables. What happens is that fibre binds itself strongly to zinc and prevents its absorption.

Cooking

Cooking can reduce the negative effects of phytic acid and fibre on zinc absorption. By the way, unlike certain vitamins, zinc cannot be destroyed by cooking at high temperatures. But, of course, large amounts of zinc can be leached out of food if you throw out the water it was cooked in. Keep the water and you keep the zinc. That's why some vegetable soups can be such excellent sources of zinc.

Refined Foods

Removing the husk from cereals is the oldest, most universal, and most efficient way of reducing the amount of zinc. 80% of the zinc in wheat is removed in the milling. Apart from other factors, the refining process is a way of protecting flour against insects and other parasites who cannot survive without zinc. See how much zinc is lost in the refining process of just two common foods: wheat flour and rice.

	mg zinc per 100g
Wholewheat flour	3.5
Whole grain rice	1.2
White flour (refined)	0.8
White (de-husked) rice	0.2

There are both pros and cons in various food processing methods. Some are able to destroy undesirable substances like phytic acid and so increase the bio-availability of zinc. On the debit side, however, techniques such as adding polyphosphates reduce the absorption of zinc.

The Answer Lies in the Soil (Or the Sea)

Whether you get your supply of zinc from animal or vegetable sources, the essential thing to know is that this mineral has its origins in the soil, or the sea. The amount of zinc in plants depends on how rich the soil is where the plants grow.

The worrying thing is that cultivated soil is becoming more and more impoverished in zinc. Though of course there are some soils which are naturally poor in zinc. The zinc in soil is in the form of soluble salts, so heavy rainfall or ice can wash the element away from the topsoil. Indeed, the small amount of zinc in the topsoil of certain regions is a result of the Ice Age.

Today, however, zinc is being robbed from soils because of modern farming techniques and the use of chemical fertilizers. Who would have thought that after half a century of annual harvests the best soils would be exhausted of zinc? This is what is happening in parts of Egypt, Iran and Iraq. Originally, these were fertile soils — but then they were farmed for centuries upon centuries. The sad thing is that in those regions where the soil is not totally exhausted, the habitual use of fertilizers — especially phosphate fertilizers — makes whatever zinc may be left in the soil as good as useless. Knowing as we do now how much people need zinc and how critical the soil is in supplying zinc, one can only be outraged at farming methods which rob zinc from the soil. Surely, sooner or later, economic considerations will have to come second to basic human needs.

The other problem is pollution in the seas where oysters — the richest food source of zinc — are harvested. Oysters come from the bottom of the sea near the coast so are exposed to pollution. The oyster is able to concentrate the bacteria and viruses in the environment thousands of times. The main risks of eating contaminated oysters are hepatitis and typhoid. Oysters also contain 3-4mg per g of cadmium, and 7-8mg per 100g of copper. The high zinc content of oysters may explain why they have long had the reputation of being an aphrodisiac; and their high price certainly makes them a luxury food. But they are not safe to eat in many parts of the world.

Could You Be Taking in Too Little Zinc?

In brief, there is a risk of taking in too little zinc if you are eating a low-protein diet, a low-energy diet, if you are a vegetarian or a vegan, or if you are eating too many refined or processed foods. Poor people are more likely to be zinc deficient than people who can afford good quality foods. Modern farming and food manufacturing techniques can be blamed for a loss of zinc in the foods which at one time had more. Careless cooking can also rob you of zinc.

4

How Much Zinc Do You Need?

How much zinc does anyone need? It sounds like a simple question. Yet the answer is not so simple — it all depends.

It depends on what you eat. It depends on what vitamin and mineral supplements you are taking. It depends on how much these nutrients are being absorbed. It depends on your genetic inheritance. It depends on your hormonal balance. It depends on your emotional stability. It depends on how old you are. It depends on whether you are male or female. It depends on where you live, and it depends on your lifestyle.

Notwithstanding these formidable factors, some public health bodies have attempted to come up with their Recommended Daily Allowances (RDAs).

In the United States, the Food and Nutrition Board of the American National Research Council published the following RDAs for zinc, according to age:

	mg
Birth to 6 months	3
6 months to one year	5
1 year to 10 years	10
Adults	15
Pregnant women	20
Breastfeeding women	25

In Canada, the authorities are incredibly precise in their recommendations:

	mg
Birth to 6 months	4
6 months to 1 year	5
1-3 years	5
4-6 years	6

From then on, the RDAs are different for men and women:

Males (years of age)	mg
7-9	7
10-12	8
13-15	10
16-18	12
19-35	10
36-50	10
Over 50	10

Females (years of age)	mg
7-9	7
10-12	9
13-15	10
16-18	11
19-35	9
36-50	9
Over 50	9
Pregnant women	12
Breastfeeding women	16

In Czechoslovakia, the authorities recommend 8mg a day for adults. In both Denmark and Italy the recommended daily intake of zinc for adults is set at 15mg as in the USA.

The DHSS in the United Kingdom has not set any recommended daily dietary allowances for zinc. In April 1979 the DHSS went on record as saying: 'Deficiency (of zinc) . . . is either rare, or associated with certain medical conditions and has not been confirmed in the United Kingdom . . .. Therefore, in the light of the present knowledge and in the context of the United Kingdom diet, recommended amounts . . . have not been set.' It is thought that the average UK diet provides 11.16mg of zinc a day, though that may be a somewhat over-optimistic estimate, and some people have estimated that figure as somewhere between 9mg and 10mg of zinc a day.

Zinc As a Trace Element

Zinc is one of the trace elements, or trace minerals. The definition of a trace element is that it occurs in the body at very low concentrations, usually less than 0.01% of the body's weight. Zinc is one of 12 trace elements which are recognized as essential for humans. In order of demonstrated need, these are:

1. Iron	4. Manganese	7. Molybdenum	10. Tin
2. Iodine	5. Zinc	8. Selenium	11. Vanadium
3. Copper	6. Cobalt	9. Chromium	12. Fluorine

The trace elements are integral components of many enzymes and some hormones in the body. They are different from the macro-elements in that they have no part to play in the structural make-up of the body (except perhaps fluoride in bones and teeth), and they are needed in far lesser amounts.

A macro-element is present in high quantities in the body and in the diet. A daily intake is normally more than 100mg. At this end of the scale are calcium, phosphorus and magnesium. At the opposite end of the scale are iodine, selenium and chromium, of which your daily need is measured in micrograms.

Just because you need more of the macro-elements does not mean they are more important to health. A deficiency of the so-called trace elements can be as damaging to your health as a deficiency of the major minerals.

Why Do Some People Need More Zinc Than Others?

As we said at the beginning of the chapter, how much zinc you need as an individual depends on a whole range of factors, including your age, sex, lifestyle and genetic make-up. But it's even more complex than that. The other nutrients — or anti-nutrients — you are eating can be important too. In fact, how much zinc you need compared to the person down the road can also depend on wider environmental issues such as methods of contraception, domestic plumbing, whether you smoke or not, and how you cook your food.

Low levels of zinc are very common in western technological societies. People who discover they have low zinc levels often ask why. Here are some questions to ask yourself.

Are you eating too much phytic acid in your diet? Have you become a vegetarian during adulthood? Are you vegan? Are you losing zinc by the way you cook your food? Are you eating too many refined and processed foods? The reasons for asking these questions are discussed in the previous chapter, but there are some less obvious questions to ask as well.

Are You Absorbing the Zinc You Are Taking?

The bio-availability of zinc is not the same in all foods containing zinc (see previous chapter). However, some people have more difficulty absorbing zinc than others, even if they are eating foods in which zinc is bio-available, or taking supplements. Zinc is absorbed in the upper part of the small intestine.

Studies in animals show that absorption becomes more efficient as dietary zinc intake declines. Though we don't know whether the efficiency of absorption is decreased when the intake goes up. Absorption in the intestines depends to some extent on what other minerals are being taken. In addition, there may be problems absorbing zinc if the person has a high histamine level, or is deficient in sulphur.

Sometimes people taking zinc supplements find that they are not absorbing one type. For example, some people do not absorb zinc orotate very well. If this seems to be happening, switching to another type often increases absorption, e.g. to zinc sulphate.

Reports from the Department of Pediatrics at the Children's

Hospital of Michigan indicate that zinc absorption is greatly enhanced by the presence of picolinic acid. This derives from the amino acid tryptophan, and is a major constituent of pancreatin. So it would be possible to take either tryptophan or pancreatin to improve the absorption of zinc.

Are You Eating Enough Essential Fatty Acids?

One reason why one person may need more zinc than another is that person's intake of essential fatty acids. If your diet is poor in essential fatty acids you will need to take more zinc. The zinc will then be able to maximize what little essential fatty acids there are. On the other hand, if your diet is very rich in essential fatty acids you will need correspondingly less zinc. In general, an average western diet is rather poor in essential fatty acids. It tends to be high in animal fats.

Essential fatty acids are called 'essential' because your body cannot make them itself — you have to eat the foods containing them. There are several essential fatty acids. The one which zinc is involved in, and which starts the ball rolling towards prostaglandins 1, is linoleic acid.

Linoleic acid is found mostly in seed oils such as sunflower seed oil or safflower seed oil. However, linoleic acid has to be in a certain form in order to be biologically active. Chemists call this the 'cis' form. The oil must not have been processed for it still to be in the 'cis' form. Heating the oil at high temperatures will make it biologically useless. Zinc is vital to help turn cis-linoleic acid into prostaglandins (see Figure 1 on page 13).

Are You Eating the Wrong Kind of Fats?

Another reason why one person may need more zinc than another is the kind of fats he is eating. When oils are refined, in particular when linoleic acid is heated at very high temperatures, the molecule of the fatty acid changes its shape. It is no longer in the 'cis' form, but has turned into what is called the 'trans' form. Trans fatty acids are useless in the metabolic process which leads to prostaglandins. Not only that, but trans fatty acids actually block the chemical reactions and work against the positive catalytic action of zinc. Put in everyday terms, this means that if you eat chips, pastries, processed oils, and the like, you are increasing your need for zinc. You need more zinc in order to get the most out of what little cis linoleic acid you are getting in your daily diet.

Are You Eating Enough of Zinc's Co-Factors?

A third reason why some people need more zinc than others is that some people are taking in more of the right 'co-factors' than others. Zinc works together with certain collaborators, known by chemists as 'co-factors'. The two particular co-factors for zinc are vitamin C and vitamin B_6. If your diet has plenty of these two vitamins, you will need less zinc than if your diet was rather low in them.

Vitamin C is found mostly in foods such as oranges and lemons, soft fruits like blackcurrants and strawberries, green vegetables and

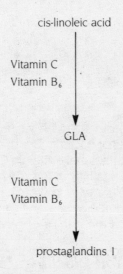

Figure 2. The co-factors of zinc

potatoes. Vitamin B_6 is found mostly in bran, wheat germ, grains, root vegetables and green leafy vegetables, Liver is the richest source of B_6 in meat. Brewer's yeast is also a rich source of this vitamin.

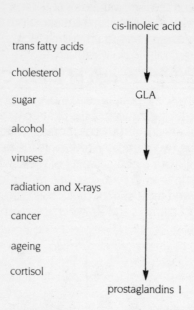

Figure 3.   The opponents of zinc

The body can synthesize its own vitamin B_6; it is probably produced by the intestinal bacteria. But this is not the case with vitamin C. Your body cannot make vitamin C for itself, and so you have to eat the foods containing it. But you have to be careful not to destroy the vitamin C in your food. It can be destroyed by refining or by heating at high temperatures, and can be lost if you throw away the water in which the fruit or vegetables were cooked.

Are You Blocking Zinc?

Another reason why some people need more zinc than others is all the blocking agents — things which can block the same reactions which zinc is trying to help. Because as well as having friendly collaborators, zinc also has opponents. Trans fatty acids are one group of blocking agents, but there are many more besides. Cholesterol is one of them; sugar is another.

Diabetes creates disturbances in the metabolism of essential fatty acids and the synthesis of prostaglandins. Alcohol interferes with all the chemical reactions to do with the synthesis of prostaglandins. Other blocking agents are radiation and X-rays. Cancer cells, too, seem to have lost their ability to go beyond GLA. Viruses can also be considered as blocking agents. Viral infections can indeed create vicious circles. Just when the immune system needs all its powers to fight against a virus, the virus blocks the synthesis of prostaglandins and so stops the immune system from being in an optimum condition to fight the viral infection.

Cortisol

Of all the blocking agents, perhaps the one which should be emphasized the most is cortisol. Cortisol is a hormone which is secreted by the adrenal gland. Cortisol not only blocks all the reactions in the metabolic pathway leading to prostaglandins, but it also inhibits the workings of the thymus. Cortisol reduces the volume of the thymus, and stops it secreting its own hormone, thymosine. So, cortisol depresses the immune system by its effects on the thymus — an organ whose functions always call for large quantities of zinc.

The type of situation which makes the level of cortisol go up is that without any way out, or without any hope — helplessness and hopelessness. The French scientist Henri Laborit called this 'inhibition of action'. People who are suffering from depression often have a high level of cortisol, and unfortunately depression is common in our modern society.

If you want to create experimental depression in animals, all you have to do is separate mother and baby. By doing this, you create a situation of helplessness. It's the same with human babies. When the basic needs of babies are not met, when they find themselves in a situation without hope and with no way out, their levels of cortisol go up at a time in their lives when they have not yet adjusted the set point levels of their basic hormones. So they get used to living with a raised level of cortisol.

This is a key to understanding the true nature of most of the so-called diseases of civilization. It is also yet another explanation why modern people need more zinc.

Are You Disturbing Your Day/Night Rhythm?

It seems that any kind of disturbance in the day/night rhythm interferes with the metabolic functions which consume a lot of zinc. This has to do with the pineal gland, a small reddish formation the size of a pea which is situated in the deepest part of the brain. It secretes the hormone melatonin. For a long time no one knew what the pineal gland was for. Descartes thought it was the seat of the soul. However, it is only recently that the pineal gland and its hormone melatonin have been understood.

There are rhythmic secretions of melatonin, reaching a maximum in the middle of the night and a minimum during the day. As a matter of interest, it takes eleven days for the pineal gland of a traveller to recover after changing time zones. The hormone melatonin encourages the synthesis of prostaglandins 1 by mobilizing its direct precursor. It plays a role in the balance between prostaglandins 1 and 2, and favours the route towards prostaglandins 1.

When you look at our modern world today, it is obvious that there are disturbances in the day/night rhythm from the time of birth onwards.

Do You Have a Good Hormonal Balance?

In fact, everything to do with your hormonal balance has an effect on the metabolism of essential fatty acids. So this means your hormonal balance has an effect on how much zinc you need too.

Insulin, which is secreted by the pancreas, is needed in these particular chemical reactions. Prolactin, the hormone which allows milk to flow in breastfeeding women, favours the synthesis of prostaglandins 1 from its direct precursor. The endorphins, which are natural opiates, have a complex action which can be either stimulating or inhibiting, depending on the specific target. In general, the stress hormones seem to have a greater tendency to block the reactions in the synthesis of prostaglandins. This is so with the adrenal hormones. Oestrogens inhibit the metabolism of unsaturated fatty acids.

The Contraceptive Pill

The pill robs women of zinc. Use of the pill brings about a mineral imbalance, especially low zinc and high copper. And oestrogen in the pill inhibits the very important metabolism of essential fatty acids. Even when a woman comes off the pill, she is still likely to be zinc deficient. If a woman gets pregnant soon after stopping the pill, she is likely to be zinc deficient at the start of her pregnancy. Some doctors and medical researchers believe that if a pregnant woman is low in zinc, the children are also likely to be zinc deficient and to start life with a mineral imbalance which they will never be able to rectify, with long-term bad effects.

Are You Taking in Minerals Which Compete with Zinc?

Another explanation for the wide range in needs for zinc is the competition between minerals. In today's world, you are likely to be taking in more minerals which compete with zinc, than zinc. If so, you need more zinc to tip the balance in favour of zinc.

Calcium

Zinc interacts with calcium in the intestinal contents where both minerals combine with phytic acid to produce an insoluble complex.

Cadmium

Cadmium is one of the heavy metals. It has the effect of taking zinc's place in chemical reactions. Cadmium is an insidious poison whose effects accumulate over the years. The more cadmium your body has in it, the more zinc you need.

The most likely sources of cadmium are cigarette smoke; the atmosphere (especially near foundries); and some foodstuffs, which can contain traces of cadmium — oysters, for example, and vegetables which have been grown in soil polluted by fertilizers containing superphosphates.

The human body has a natural mechanism for protecting itself against cadmium. This is by means of a protein which binds with cadmium called metallothionein. But the best way to protect yourself against too much cadmium is to increase your intake of zinc.

Copper

How much zinc you need also depends on how much copper you are taking in. The body needs small amounts of copper to be able to synthesize haemoglobin, the pigment in red blood cells which carries oxygen. In practice, an average diet always has enough copper in it; if anything, it usually has too much.

When the level of copper in the blood goes too high it interferes with the absorption of zinc. If this happens, more zinc is needed. This is very likely precisely what is happening with people living in the modern world. Man only needs about 2mg of copper a day, but nowadays he is more likely taking in between 3-5mg. Why is this?

Most people are ingesting more copper than they need due to the use of copper pipes in plumbing, particularly in pipes used for drinking water. Small amounts of copper can also get into foodstuffs when you cook with copper pots and pans which have lost their chrome coating. This could also happen if you keep liquids in any copper container. Some insecticides contain copper, and this can get into food. Some chemical additives also contain copper. For example the additive E141 is a complex of copper and chlorophyl which is used as a colouring agent in some sweets and certain cheeses.

In addition to copper in foodstuffs, women who use copper intra-uterine devices as a contraceptive will also be absorbing more copper than they actually need.

The best way to counteract too much copper is to increase your intake of zinc.

Are You Taking In Too Much Lead?

If you live in a city and drive a car, your lead level may be higher than somebody's who lives in the country and doesn't regularly breathe in exhaust fumes. If so, you need more zinc — because zinc is an essential nutrient for getting rid of toxic metals from the body.

Lead is a toxic metal. Lead levels in our modern environment are probably 500 to 1,000 times what they were in prehistoric times, and most of the increase has happened during this century. Evidence of lead pollution can be found all over the world in samples of soil and snow. The lead in petrol is mostly to blame. This began in 1921, when Midgley discovered that lead improved a car's performance. Lead from car exhaust fumes, inhaled directly or by settling on foodstuffs, can particularly affect children — lead toxicity can affect children's IQ, their learning ability and their behaviour.

Only the USSR has really done something about the lead problem, and in 1960 prohibited lead in petrol. But in western countries it is only very recently that a start has been made to either reduce or withdraw lead from petrol. Very late in the day, western car manufacturers are taking a leaf out of the Japanese car manufacturers' book — Japanese cars are designed to work without lead in petrol.

An atmosphere polluted by car exhaust fumes is not the only way we can take in too much lead. It can also come from the food we eat and the water we drink, since there are still lead pipes in use. Due to lead pollution on such a widespread scale there is an increasing need for whatever nutrients can reduce the absorption and toxicity of lead.

Zinc as a De-toxifier

Zinc is very important for its ability to de-toxify lead. Studies have shown that zinc, together with vitamin C, can reduce blood lead levels in men working in factories making lead batteries.

Are You Taking In Too Much Mercury?

The problems posed by mercury — another heavy metal — are not very different from those of lead — although mercury pollution is not on the same scale. A variety of industries tip mercury into rivers and lakes; algae transform it into organic by-products which are toxic. At each stage of the food chain the concentration of organic mercury increases. So the fish which eat the algae have a concentration of mercury which is 100 times higher. With some types of big fish, such as swordfish, it has reached such a level that they are no longer edible.

Mercury—Amalgam Fillings in Dentistry

There are some dentists who believe that in some people the mercury in fillings is getting into the body and is implicated in some neurological symptoms, perhaps in multiple sclerosis. One possible remedy is to have the fillings removed. But a less drastic one (removal of mercury—amalgam fillings has its own dangers) is to step up your intake of the de-toxifying nutrients — zinc and vitamin C in particular.

Two Quick and Simple Ways to Detect a Zinc Deficiency

White Marks on the Nails

Doctor Carl Pfeiffer was the first to show the real significance of little white spots on the nails, especially in children and adolescents, but also in some adults. Doctors call these little white spots 'leuconychies'. Some people have thought that the white spots were calcium deposits, but there is no evidence for this. In 1956, Muerkcke noticed that these white marks on the nails appeared frequently in diseases where the level of albumin in the plasma was low, especially kidney diseases and cirrhosis of the liver. Later, Pfeiffer concluded that the white spots, or marks, were signs of zinc deficiency. As a large part of zinc is bonded to albumin, a sizeable deficit in albumin often goes together with a deficit in zinc.

However, the fact that some unquestionable deficits in zinc can happen without any lowering of albumin in the serum leads one to a quite different interpretation. The nails grow about 3mm a month and completely renew themselves about every 6 months. So it is possible to pinpoint the exact period when someone suffered a temporary shortage of zinc by estimating the date when the white spot or mark happened. Sometimes this corresponds in an obvious way to a period of fasting among some religious communities.

The Taste Test

The taste test is brilliant in its simplicity. It makes use of the fact that someone who is short of zinc will not be able to taste things properly, including the metallic taste of zinc itself. Subjects are asked to taste a solution made up of 1g of zinc sulphate in a litre of distilled water. The results of the taste test fall into four categories:

(i)   No particular taste sensation after keeping the solution in the mouth for about 10 seconds.
(ii) Only being able to taste something after a few seconds.
(iii) A distinctive taste is perceived immediately, but it is not a nasty one.
(iv) A very nasty, distinctive taste is perceived straightaway.

Categories (i) and (ii) show a lack of zinc. Subjects are considered good candidates for zinc supplements. Categories (iii) and (iv) show no lack of zinc.

This taste test is used by Professor Derek Bryce-Smith at Reading University, and home testing kits are available from a health products company by mail order.

One day, simple tests like this might be typical of the kind of real advances to be made in medicine when the diseases of civilization are better understood.

How Do You Measure Zinc Status in the Body?

How much zinc you need is difficult to evaluate because at the moment there is no perfect indicator of an individual's zinc status. Some people believe they have found the right technique, but there is considerable disagreement about how good such techniques really are. A variety of methods have been put forward.

Zinc Levels in the Plasma
The level of zinc in the plasma varies according to the time of day, how recently you ate a meal, and to whether you have recently been subjected to stressful events. So plasma levels of zinc cannot really be taken as an accurate way of testing the body's zinc status. Plasma tests usually give results of between 70 and 120μg per 100ml.

Hair Analysis
There has been a raging controversy about the benefits of using hair analysis to measure zinc (and other minerals). Some people are convinced it works, while others are not so sure. Hair analysis has many attractions as a diagnostic test; it is quick and easy to take a sample of hair, but not so easy to analyse.

The concentration of minerals in the hair is five times that in the blood. Hair contains on average 125 - 225μg per gram, but the exact measurement of zinc from hair analysis seems to be open to a margin of error. Hair reflects contamination in the environment, and the use of particular shampoos. The results can also depend on how fast the hair grows. So, hair analysis would seem not to be the ideal way of assessing someone's zinc status.

Urine Testing
The level of zinc in urine is not significant. If you test urine for zinc, all it will show is the amount of zinc lost in the urine. But it won't

show the amount of zinc in the body as a whole. About 400 - 600μg of zinc is normally excreted in the urine every day. In some conditions of zinc deficiency, a small amount of zinc is excreted in the urine, but in others the opposite can be the case. So, urine is not necessarily a good method of detecting zinc deficiency.

Most zinc is excreted from the body in the stools. If the stools are analysed, one can find zinc which has not been absorbed by the intestine and zinc which has been secreted by pancreatic and intestinal juices. Some zinc is lost from the body in sweat, though the loss is only significant when it goes above 1mg per litre.

Leucocyte Testing

Another way to find out someone's zinc status is to test the level of zinc in the white blood cells. This is a good indicator of the level of zinc in the tissues generally. The best way is to test the polymorphonuclear leucocytes. This method was suggested by Jones and Keeling in London at the end of the 1970s. Not much blood is needed for this particular test, nor does it involve any great technical difficulties.

The Sweat Test

It seems that the best reflection of the body's zinc status is the sweat test. It was devised by biochemist Dr John Howard of the Biolab Medical Unit in Weymouth Street, London. A small absorbent pad, about the size of a sticky plaster, is placed on the person's back. The pad is made of a special, highly absorbent, material. After about an hour the pad is taken off and mixed with 1% nitric acid which extracts metals from the pad. A highly sophisticated machine called an Atomic Absorption Spectrophotometer is then used to analyse very precisely the trace elements extracted from the sweat pad. At the time of writing the Biolab was the only place able to offer the sweat test, and it is quite expensive.

The Taste Test
See page 45.

Conclusion

Our analysis of the factors which influence how much zinc you need leads to the conclusion that man living in western industrialized societies is constantly on the brink of being deficient in zinc. A comparison between modern man and the hunter-gatherer of prehistoric times shows this very clearly. Genetically, the hunter-gatherer is our contemporary. In the course of his life the hunter-gatherer did not ingest the amount of cadmium, copper, lead and mercury that we do now.

The fact that prehistoric man was solidly integrated into a community meant that he was probably protected against depression, which is so common nowadays in our world of greater social isolation. Put another way, his lifestyle was such that he was protected against a chronically high level of cortisol.

When the hunter-gatherer ate meat, it was wild game — very different from the meat of intensively reared farm animals fed on grain. The protein/fat ratio was very high, and the fat was very rich in unsaturated fatty acids. Nowadays meat is high in saturated fat. And, needless to say, there were no refined oils in those days.

As for the vegetables eaten by the hunter-gatherer, they were more varied in the days before the culture of cereals was well organized. Since the advent of agriculture, cereals have yielded more starch for less protein. In prehistoric times, it was the other way round.

Compared with modern man, the hunter-gatherer had a lower need for zinc, and at the same time had almost as high an intake. It is worth keeping this in mind when trying to assess basic human needs.

Huge Zinc Deficiency States: Acrodermatitis Enteropathica and Dwarfism

It is worthwhile examining some huge deficiency states of zinc in both animals and man where the consequences are very severe so that one can be better at detecting zinc deficiency states which are less obvious.

There is an animal model of massive zinc deficiency. It affects a variety of calves which belong to the breed of Black Pied Danish Cattle. This particular kind of calf, known as 'A-46' is a mutant of the breed. What is peculiar about the A-46 calf is that for some reason it is totally incapable of using zinc and is in a state of being massively deficient — a condition which is incompatible with survival.

A study about these calves was published in 1971. One of the most striking observations of the researchers was that the thymus did not develop at all in these calves. This confirms the importance of zinc in all the immune functions, in particular the functions of the thymus.

However, one cannot draw too many conclusions from animal models like this because man is of course different, and the metabolic chains do not work in exactly the same way from one mammal to another. The cat, for example, cannot make gammalinolenic acid from linoleic acid, whereas man and other mammals can do this thanks to a chemical reaction involving zinc.

In any case, this animal model is completely eclipsed by the existence of a human one; a genetic disease which involves a huge deficiency of zinc due to problems in being able to use whatever zinc is in the food.

The first description of this disease is all the more interesting because it was not in any way influenced by some theories which have become popular since 1943, when a paper was published by Niels Danbolt and Karl Closs. It is interesting to note that these men were dermatologists; people whose interest is centred on diseases of the skin. The name they gave to this illness is highly significant: Acrodermatitis Enteropathica. This suggests that it first appeared as a skin disease, especially localized at the extremities. The name also suggests that it is an illness involving absorption from the intestines.

Acrodermatitis Enteropathica

They wrote a detailed picture of this illness, describing two cases. This description is still the best document of reference. Alongside the text there are some photos to illustrate these two cases, a baby and a young child. These show exactly what the local pustules look like, especially around the orifices and the protruding parts of the head, trunk, and extremities. You can see that the fingertips are swollen and the nails atrophied. The children are completely bald; the eyelids are closed; and one of the children displays a tongue covered in tiny buds. The text describes symptoms of diarrhoea with fatty, foul-smelling stools.

The authors of this description point out that the symptoms appear at infancy or in early childhood. It has since been confirmed that the beginning of this disease corresponds to the time of weaning. It is a chronic disease which evolves in a series of relapses and remissions. During a flare-up, the patient displays behaviour which is similar to that of a schizophrenic. Growth is considerably retarded, as well as brain growth.

As they were writing about this disease in 1943, it is not surprising that the authors did not say anything about the thymus. At that time, no one knew about all the functions of the thymus and no one thought about measuring its size or looking at it closely in an examination. Also at that time no one knew how important zinc was either. No one guessed that zinc might be involved in the genesis of this disease.

No treatment worked, despite trials with different vitamins, liver extracts, hormones, a variety of drugs, and a gluten-free diet. The disease was nearly always fatal. At the end of 1953 it was noticed by chance that these patients could be helped considerably by anti-malarial drugs such as diodoquine, although no one understood why.

It was only in 1974 and 1975 that the first spectacular cures were reported using zinc sulphate and that the claim could be made that acrodermatitis enteropathica was a condition where the body was unable to use zinc.

What struck the doctors who first used zinc for this disease was not just that the treatment worked, but that it was so fast. It did this for every symptom, not just the obvious ones but also the more subtle ones which could only be detected in the laboratory. In 1975 a team in Denver, Colorado did a very detailed study which showed that from the first 24 hours of treatment there was a marked improvement; and a complete remission could be achieved in four days.

Once they knew that zinc worked, the penny dropped as to why the anti-malarial drugs had worked — these drugs can bind themselves to zinc, and guarantee that zinc will get carried along. Nowadays it is thought that acrodermatitis enteropathica is partly due to the absence of a substance in the intestine whose role is to bind to zinc and allow its absorption. Despite this, large amounts of zinc seem to be able to overcome this defect.

Dwarfism

For a long time, no one could understand why some males in Iran had stunted growth. These dwarfs lived in villages where the staple diet was unleavened bread. At puberty, these dwarfs had only infantile genitals, and their IQ was low. In that part of the world, the soil had been cultivated for several centuries and was poor in zinc. Here was the clue.

A scientist by the name of Prasad did some spectacular work with these Iranian dwarfs. When they ate a diet enriched with zinc they developed normal sexual function. If the boys were still under 20 years old and their bones were still growing, they could achieve an astounding increase in height of about 10cms on the zinc therapy.

The knowledge which scientists gained about zinc from these two states of huge deficiency paved the way for research into other areas.

6

Fertility, Pregnancy and Birth

Probably the most exciting area concerning zinc is reproduction. Zinc seems to be vital for fertility and for the normal growth of a healthy foetus. We are still at a stage of needing more solid research before one can make any hard and fast statements about such topics as infertility in males, foetal growth retardation, foetal malformations, miscarriages and stillbirths, but, from what we know so far, zinc promises to be a vital element — perhaps *the* vital element — in these conditions which can cause so much human unhappiness.

Infertility in Men

Zinc is vital for the normal development of the male sex organs. This was shown to be the case in the Iranian dwarfs (see previous chapter). If there is a lack of zinc the male sex organs do not mature properly. Zinc is needed by the testes, the seminal vessels and the prostate. Sperm is also loaded with zinc — it has been claimed that each ejaculation corresponds to a loss of 1mg of zinc.

Zinc is a good indicator of fertility: the zinc concentration in semen corresponds to the number of sperm in fertile men. There is some evidence from Sweden that subfertility in males can be treated by giving extra zinc.

Pregnancy

The authorities in the USA reckon that pregnant women need 20mg of zinc a day — 5mg more than an adult woman who is not pregnant.

If an average adult is thought to be taking in only about 10mg of zinc a day, this means that pregnant women may be taking in only half the recommended amount of zinc. How much zinc a pregnant woman should have, and whether or not she needs or should take zinc supplements, is a matter of heated controversy among scientists.

Foresight, the British group who promote pre-conceptual care, work with scientists such as Professor Derek Bryce-Smith from the Department of Organic Chemistry at Reading University. He is a great believer in zinc supplements for all pregnant women. He says: 'Zinc is the most prevalent nutrient lacking in pregnancy.' Pregnancy places special demands on the mother, and zinc is vital for the growing foetus. A lot of attention has been paid to folic acid, and zinc is needed for the absorption of folic acid during pregnancy.

The microbial activity of the amniotic fluid is dependent on the level of zinc. Professor Bryce-Smith, and others, believe that zinc in pregnancy, from the time of conception, is so important that a lack of it is implicated in certain foetal abnormalities, stillbirths, low birth-weight and other problems affecting babies and children. He believes that if the mother is zinc-deficient during her pregnancy, the baby will be born zinc-deficient — with long-term consequences.

However, this view is not shared by Dr Peter Aggett, Co-ordinator for the Centre for Study of Metabolism of Trace Elements at the University of Aberdeen. Dr Aggett thinks zinc supplementation in pregnancy is probably unnecessary. Dr Aggett says: 'The provision of zinc supplements has not been found to have clear cut beneficial effects on foetal outcome or the quality of the pregnancy and labour. Also, since the most critical period of foetal development precedes the usual stage at which pregnancy is diagnosed, supplements given subsequently would have no effect on most developmental abnormalities. Thus, the need for zinc supplementation in normal healthy pregnant women is, to say the least, questionable.'

While the controversy continues it would seem perfectly safe for any woman who favours the *Foresight* way of thinking to take zinc supplements of up to 30mg a day from the time she starts to *think* about getting pregnant.

In any case, taking zinc supplements would probably be more useful and less harmful than iron tablets, which are prescribed routinely though there are no studies to back this up. Too much iron will upset the mineral balance and get in the way of the absorption of zinc. However, zinc on its own can also create a mineral imbalance — particularly by lowering manganese. So a zinc supplement should be taken together with manganese.

Animal Studies on Zinc and Pregnancy

In animal studies, zinc deprivation has been found to cause a wide spectrum of abnormalities during pregnancy. Diets low in zinc resulted in miscarriages early in pregnancy, and foetal abnormalities. At the end of a pregnancy, zinc-deficient diets caused delayed or prolonged labour, death of the newborn during labour or shortly afterwards, and poor maternal instincts in those mothers whose offspring survived.

Vets and stockbreeders have confirmed these findings. For fifty years, breeders in New Zealand had to face 'the sulky cow syndrome'. Cows with this disease were very weak, had a poor appetite, developed eczema on the tail and fell into deep lethargy after calving. Some cows died at the end of their pregnancy. Others had a difficult labour and delivery and gave birth to either a weak or a dead calf.

It was discovered that 'the sulky cow syndrome' was due to a lack of zinc brought about by a fungal toxin in the grass of some grazing pastures. A New Zealand farmer by the name of Mrs Gladys Reid noted that a coffee cup of zinc sulphate (about 5g) put even the illest animals back on their feet, and the cows could give birth to healthy calves.

The studies in which experimental animals were deliberately deprived of zinc cannot be compared with the human situation. It seems that, in the animal studies, the levels of zinc used were far lower than those in women living in the western world. Also, the experiments were conducted in such a way that the pregnant animals were not able to use whatever zinc they already had in their bodies and pass it on to their babies.

Even so, these animal studies do have some lessons for us and it would seem a good idea to take a serious view of any lack of zinc in pregnant women, and to carry out proper studies. However, such studies are difficult, as many factors are involved, as well as ethical issues.

Studies of Pregnant Women Low in Zinc Who Had Normal Babies

Also, there have been some studies of women who were known to be taking low levels of zinc during their pregnancy but who gave birth to perfectly normal babies. There is a great deal to be learned from pregnant women about our powers of adaptation and how poorly people living in the modern world adapt to their environment.

In my work in a small French hospital, I had the opportunity of seeing many immigrants, North Africans in particular. They mostly came from the lower socio-economic groups. Generally, their diet is poor in proteins of animal origin, and certainly poor in zinc. Even so, the women usually give birth to normal weight, healthy babies.

The birth is usually easy, on condition that it takes place in a small room which looks nothing like a typical delivery room, where the atmosphere is intimate, the light is dim, and there are no men. North African women are particularly disturbed and inhibited by conventional hospitals with their delivery beds.

At the same time, I also had the opportunity of seeing many western women who had decided to become vegetarian as adults. Mostly these women came from families who were comfortably-off. More often than could have happened just by chance, these women had low birth-weight babies, or else their babies died still inside the uterus. Their births were often particularly difficult. All too often, these women had taken iron supplements during the pregnancy — but only iron supplements. This doubled their chances of being low in zinc — first because of their vegetarian diet when they had not developed the phytase enzyme to get the most zinc from their food; and secondly because supplements of iron create a greater need for zinc.

The zinc status of a pregnant woman cannot be taken out of context of her culture. The women who had switched to vegetarianism in adulthood had been used to a good zinc intake up till then from the meat they used to eat. So their bodies find it hard to adapt to a lower intake of zinc. This lower intake might be the same as a woman who has always been vegetarian, but for her this level of zinc is normal, not abnormal.

For example, there were some studies done with Asian women whose traditional diet is vegetarian. The results confirmed the extraordinary adaptability of these women. The Gujaratis in India have a zinc intake of about 7.6mg a day. When they come to the United Kingdom some of them stick to their vegetarian habit (59%), while others develop the new habit of meat-eating.

As might have been expected, these studies showed that these particular women needed very little zinc. The six women in the studies who had less than 5mg of zinc a day gave birth to normal-weight babies. What seems to be important is not the number of milligrams of zinc during the pregnancy, but the diet the woman had been accustomed to since infancy.

As there have been so few studies, one can only put forward hypotheses as to why some western women are poor at adapting once they have been used to a diet rich in proteins of animal origin. The studies which have tried to establish correlations between the level of zinc in the blood of pregnant women and the length and difficulty of labour are difficult to interpret. This is because the blood level is not a good indicator of zinc status, and the blood zinc level drops anyway during pregnancy as a result of the increased volume of blood flowing through the pregnant woman's body which dilutes zinc (and other) levels. This is why one should not give undue weight to the studies by Jameson on some Swedish women which showed a correlation between low levels of zinc in the blood and the length and difficulty of childbirth; or to studies conducted in Spain which established a correlation between the blood zinc level of the mother and the contractility of the uterus.

Perhaps more weight should be given to the studies by Meadows in the United Kingdom which revealed a correlation between a low level of zinc in the white blood cells and low birth-weight babies.

Low Birth-Weight Babies and Zinc

There was a recent study involving 100 babies born in Barnsley, Yorkshire. The researchers took 100 obstetrically normal births and analysed various tissues for some specific minerals and trace elements. They wanted to see what elements were consistent with normal foetal development; and at the same time what elements (or lack of them) were consistent with abnormal foetal development. Of all the tissues they analysed (including maternal pubic hair, whole blood from the umbilical cord and the baby's hair) only the placenta was a good indicator.

The researchers (Professor Bryce-Smith, Dr Watson and Dr Neil Ward) found a link between low placental zinc and low birth-weight. The placental zinc was low in babies weighing less than 3000g at birth. There was a progressive increase in the zinc/copper ratio as the birth weight increased. Cadmium and lead were highest in the low birth-weight babies. All these results were statistically significant.

Smoking During Pregnancy: Cadmium and Low Birth-Weight

In the Barnsley study, the researchers found that cadmium was significantly elevated in the placentas of smoking mothers. Smoking mothers had the lowest birth-weight babies. 'Passive' smokers — women who breathed in other people's cigarette smoke during their pregnancy — had lower birth-weight babies than non-smokers. In the study, only one baby weighing more than 3,500g was born to a mother who smoked.

The researchers found that the more cadmium there was in the placenta, the smaller was the baby's head when they measured the circumference. When the baby's head circumference measured less than 34cms they found a significant lack of zinc in the placenta. Cadmium is a zinc antagonist.

Foetal Abnormalities, Stillbirths and Zinc

Once a woman knows she is pregnant, the first question on her mind is: 'Will the baby be all right?' There is as yet no hard data about minerals and birth outcome. However, the frequency of some malformations seems to be strongly influenced by the mother's diet at the time of conception and the beginning of the pregnancy. This is particularly so in the case of defects in the head and the spinal cord; anencephaly and spina bifida. The few babies who survive these malformations are terribly handicapped. Worse, when a woman gives birth to a baby with spina bifida or anencephaly, her chances of having another baby with the same problems are increased ten times.

Without claiming they have what amounts to scientific evidence yet, there are some scientists who believe very strongly indeed that zinc is the most vital element during pregnancy and that the finger can be pointed to a lack of zinc in certain foetal abnormalities, some stillbirths and other anomalies affecting babies and children.

Dr Neil Ward has made a study of spina bifida in South Wales, where the condition is very common. Of all the elements he tested, he found a deficit only in zinc.

With stillborn babies, there is the hypothesis that in some cases there is a massive accumulation of zinc in the developing baby, but some mechanism in the baby causes all the zinc to be locked up in the liver, so that it is not available for protein metabolism.

It may be that zinc is indeed vital to have a healthy baby. But no one knows for certain yet which vitamins and minerals play an essential role. So at the moment it is too early to state categorically that zinc can help prevent malformations in human babies. But it looks like a hope for the future.

Pica (Abnormal Food Fads During Pregnancy)

It is perhaps something of a joke to think of pregnant women hankering after bizarre things during their pregnancy, things they would perhaps not normally ever eat, such as shoe polish. It is now believed that pica represents a mineral deficiency, and that a woman will crave foods which actually contain the missing mineral, even though she may not realize it. Zinc is often found to be the missing mineral in women with bizarre food cravings during pregnancy.

Miscarriages

Dr Carl Pfeiffer believes that a lack of zinc and vitamin B_6 may be responsible for miscarriages — particularly of boys. This is because the male foetus needs more zinc due to the zinc which goes into the male sex organs. He reports many cases of families where there are only girl children, and where the mother has miscarried only boys. When he has tested these mothers, he has found them to be zinc and B_6 deficient.

Post-Natal Depression

Doctors who specialize in nutritional medicine are now suggesting that the best remedy is to eat the placenta after delivery, as the placenta is very rich in zinc and other elements. Many of them believe that post-natal depression is quite simply a zinc deficiency, and this is because the zinc level in the mother drops two to three days before delivery, and the zinc is transferred to the baby. When mothers have been given zinc supplements after the birth, either from placenta or more conventional supplements, the post-natal depression goes away like magic, say the reports. The suggestion has been mooted that health supplement manufacturers should start making freeze-dried placenta tablets.

Toxaemia in Pregnancy (Pre-eclampsia)

Toxaemia, sometimes better known as pre-eclampsia, can sometimes happen at the end of a pregnancy. Protein suddenly appears in the urine; the blood-pressure goes worryingly high; and the ankles, fingers and other parts of the body swell up. In the worst cases, this ends in eclampsia, or a fit, which can put the mother's life in danger. Some babies do not survive toxaemia and die in the womb. Others are born weak, and look like 'spider babies', very thin but of normal height.

Even today, pre-eclampsia is still an enigma. No one is certain quite what causes it, or how to treat it other than complete rest. Over the years a variety of measures have been put forward to avoid and treat this common condition; and when you closely compare all of them, some clues begin to take shape. Zinc is just one of the many pieces of the jigsaw of pre-eclampsia.

The first of these measures was a strict milk diet. In 1900 Professor Pinard, working in a Paris maternity hospital, decided to assess the progress made by obstetrics during the nineteenth century. For him, one of the great achievements had been the prevention of pre-eclampsia by a strict milk diet. The results indeed do show that this strict milk diet prevented eclamptic fits, with 100% of women having no eclamptic fit on this regime.

The champion of the second method to avoid and treat pre-eclampsia is the American doctor Tom Brewer. He has spent his life fighting to show that a high protein diet, rich in meat, eggs, and dairy produce as well as in calories, salt, vitamins and minerals, was the key to preventing toxaemia. He based this on his personal observation of thousands of pregnant women.

Tom Brewer denounced all the dangerous methods used by doctors, such as weight loss, a salt-free diet, and the use of diuretic drugs. He drew an eloquent parallel between deaths from toxaemia in pregnancy and deaths from pellagra in the USA between 1900 and 1958. Without doubt, pellagra is a disease of malnutrition, caused primarily by a lack of nicotinic acid or niacine, one of the B group vitamins. Whenever there is a lack of nicotinic acid, it suggests that there is a lack of high quality proteins, a lack of zinc and a lack of the B vitamins in general. In the same way, one could also draw a parallel between toxaemia in pregnancy and beriberi. Beriberi is also without doubt a disease of malnutrition, attributed to a lack of the B vitamins, B_1 in particular. It is a disease which can happen to people who only eat refined rice. This particular parallel was noticed in Hong Kong during the Second World War.

A third proposal in the prevention and treatment of toxaemia in pregnancy is evening primrose oil. A team in France prescribes evening primrose oil for women at risk of developing toxaemia.

Evening primrose oil is rich in unsaturated fatty acids. It is almost unique in containing gammalinolenic acid (GLA), an almost direct precursor of prostaglandins 1. It is still too early to know whether evening primrose oil works in preventing toxaemia, but some people consider it to be theoretically promising.

The fourth way being used in the prevention of toxaemia seems at first glance to have nothing to do with the previous three. It is aspirin, in tiny doses. A team in Paris gave doses of 150mg a day to a group of at-risk women at the end of the first three months of pregnancy. These doctors prescribed the aspirin together with a drug called 'persantine' which has the reputation of preventing the platelets in the blood from sticking together. Another team in Holland gave pregnant women a lower dose of aspirin, 60mg, beginning at the end of the second trimester. Both these teams seem to have succeeded in lowering the incidence of pre-eclampsia.

What can all these different methods possibly have in common? On the face of it, they all seem quite different from each other: one says nothing but milk; the next says a high protein diet; the next suggests evening primrose oil; the other one says aspirin.

But, in fact, there is a common link between these apparently different methods. They all encourage the synthesis of certain prostaglandins, rather than others, and at the same time they reinforce the immune system. For example, it is known that aspirin blocks thromboxane, which is a variety of prostaglandins 2. Evening primrose oil contains GLA, a precursor of prostaglandins 1. If you take evening primrose oil, it's a short cut to making prostaglandins 1 and it overcomes some of the disturbances often found in the metabolism of linoleic acid.

Pre-eclampsia and Zinc

A diet which is rich in animal proteins, and a strict milk diet have certain things in common: they both provide high quality protein, and at the same time they both provide a good amount of *zinc* — which is an essential catalyst in the synthesis of prostaglandins 1.

Conventional doctors, who are so used to using drugs, would

put aspirin at the top. However, aspirin does cross the placenta and can cause haemorrhage in the foetus, so one has to be sceptical about such a risky way. It is also rather simplistic to use a drug which stops the platelets from bunching up together. After all, this is hardly a phenomenon which could be described as the prime mover of this illness.

So what is the best way to prevent and treat pre-eclampsia? Forward-thinking doctors, the ones who belong to 'nouvelle medicine' are likely to be attracted to the dietary approaches. If they prescribe supplements, evening primrose oil is likely to be one of them. However, if they want to be sure of maintaining the synthesis of prostaglandins 1, it would be a good idea to ensure a good ration of the catalysts which aid this synthesis — zinc in particular.

At the moment, there do not appear to be any large-scale studies which are evaluating the role of zinc in the prevention of pre-eclampsia. However, if evening primrose oil does turn out to be efficient, then zinc would make it even more so, the two of them working together.

Hyperactive Children, Allergic Conditions, Autism, Dyslexia and Learning Difficulties

Hyperactive Children

The origins of hyperactivity in children may well be traced back to before the child is even conceived. The mineral status of the mother at the time of conception is now thought to have long-term consequences for the child. If the mother-to-be is deficient in zinc at the time she conceives a baby, the baby could become hyperactive — in some cases while still in the womb. There have been cases where symptoms of hyperactivity started as early as 18 weeks in the womb.

There could be several reasons for the mother-to-be being zinc deficient. If she had been on the contraceptive pill, this would have lowered her zinc status. If she smoked, the cadmium from the cigarette smoke would have acted as a zinc antagonist. An excess of lead from car exhaust fumes, or an excess of aluminium from cookware, would have similar effects. Eating refined and processed foods would fail to provide the necessary amount of zinc — 83% of zinc is lost in white bread. Vegetarian or vegan diets might also be short of zinc.

Some doctors specializing in nutritional medicine believe that it may be possible to predict hyperactivity in a newborn baby if the placenta is analysed. A shortage of zinc in the placenta would be one of the indicators; a shortage of magnesium is another important one. Zinc deficiency in pregnancy may be associated with other defects in the child, such as allergies, dyslexia, autism or learning difficulties, which could develop later on into delinquency.

Nutritional Deficiencies in Hyperactive Children

When hyperactive children have their hair analysed for minerals, a common picture is a deficiency in magnesium, zinc, manganese, and chromium, and the Hyperactive Children's Support Group, a very active self-help group, recommends that, as an immediate action such nutritional deficiencies should be corrected. To achieve this supplements of these minerals should be given, along with the B vitamins, vitamins A, C, D, E, calcium, selenium, cobalt and essential fatty acids (evening primrose oil). Once the missing vitamins and minerals are replaced in the child, there is often a dramatic improvement. They sleep better, and are less hyperactive. Like *Foresight*, the HACSG believes that the best prevention for hyperactivity would be to get the diet right of mothers-to-be *before* they get pregnant.

Zinc is an important co-factor in the metabolism of essential fatty acids. Hyperactive and allergic children may be unable to convert essential fatty acids inside their bodies because they lack sufficient cis-linoleic acid or the necessary co-factors — zinc, vitamin C and some of the B vitamins.

Hyperactivity is more common in boys than girls, and this may be due to the greater need of the male sex organs for zinc.

Food Additives, Hyperactivity and Zinc

The finger has been pointed at artificial flavours and colours as the guilty parties in hyperactivity. The colouring agent tartrazine, E102, used in many yellow and orange-coloured drinks and confectionery, is often singled out as being especially harmful to hyperactive children.

Dr Ben Feingold, the American doctor who is known for the Feingold Diet for hyperactive children, has had a good deal of success by removing all salicylates, artificial flavours and colours from the diet of such children.

The reason why these artificial flavours and colours have such a dramatic effect on hyperactive children has now become clear. Salicylates, benzoates and tartrazine (as well as phytate) act as chelating agents. A chelator is something which latches or grabs onto something else. In the case of salicylates, benzoates and tartrazine they chelate with essential trace elements and interfere with their absorption. Zinc is one of those so affected.

It is known that after taking orange cordial containing tartrazine there is a massive drop in the plasma zinc of hyperactive children. Even worse, the absorption of copper and lead is thought to be increased by salicylates and tartrazine.

According to Dr Feingold, the body may also detoxify additives by coating them with zinc, and then excreting them. This means that the body's reserves of zinc and other protective nutrients are being squandered.

Once the child is low in zinc (and/or manganese) it can become more susceptible to the noxious effects of metals such as lead, copper, cadmium and aluminium. There is a heavy metal burden in hyperactive children. In any case, young people are more susceptible to toxic elements than adults. A recent study showed that lead and cadmium levels were significantly high in a group of hyperactive boys; these children also being zinc deficient.

The Link Between Pre-Menstrual Syndrome and Hyperactive Children

One of the leading doctors specializing in nutritional medicine, Dr Stephen Davies, has found a connection between pre-menstrual syndrome and hyperactivity in children. Nearly all hyperactive children have mothers who suffer from the pre-menstrual syndrome.

One nutritional approach to the treatment of pre-menstrual syndrome is evening primrose oil, together with the co-factors of zinc, vitamin C, magnesium and vitamins B_6 and nicotinamide (also known as niacin).

Although zinc is important, Dr Davies believes that the most important element in this link between PMS and hyperactivity is magnesium. When testing hyperactive children at the Biolab, of which Dr Davies is a director, they have repeatedly found a deficiency in magnesium as well as in zinc.

Allergic Conditions (Eczema, Asthma, Allergies, Hayfever)

The increase in incidences of eczema, asthma and allergies amongst the present generation of children may be due in part to a change in nutrition and an increase in environmental pollutants. However, the causes are probably much deeper than this; from what we know about allergies the first thing we should think of is the period of infant feeding.

Similar causes to those which result in hyperactive children are thought to be implicated. Children may be more prone to these allergic conditions if their mothers smoked. Smoking is known to increase levels of cadmium and lead and decrease the levels of zinc, vitamins C and E and the B complex of vitamins.

Some studies also show that a woman who was on the contraceptive pill is more likely to produce an allergic child. The pill lowers the body's zinc, manganese, vitamins B_6, B_2, B_{12} and vitamin C. By increasing the excretion of B_6 in the urine (zinc teams up with B_6) a zinc deficiency also reduces the level of nicotinamide.

In a woman who both smoked and was on the pill, the nutritional profile would be even worse. If such a woman got pregnant without correcting her nutritional deficiencies, her child would stand a risk of being more prone to allergies. This is because some essential nutrients, including zinc, are needed for the production of enzymes necessary to metabolize food correctly, and for optimal adrenal function.

Treating Allergic Conditions Nutritionally

The child may react badly to certain foods (such as wheat and milk). The first step is to identify the foods and cut them out of the diet, but a supplement of minerals and vitamins will help the healing process. The nutrients needed most are zinc, vitamin A, vitamin C, the B complex of vitamins, manganese, calcium and evening primrose oil. This will help both enzyme activity, and to get rid of lead from the body. Together with methianine 500mg and phenytoin 100mg, these nutrients are thought to have an anti-histamine effect.

These nutritional supplements have been found to work well in children with allergic conditions, especially those who suffer from abnormal thirst, and who come from 'atopic' families (families where 'atopic' conditions such as eczema, asthma, hayfever, and allergies already exist.)

Dyslexia

In a recent study, where a group of 40 dyslexic children were given the Sweat Test at the Biolab in London, every single one of them was found to be zinc-deficient. The results showed that the highest zinc level in the test group was lower than the lowest zinc level in normal children as a control, who were matched for age, sex and class.

Although this does not mean that zinc actually causes dyslexia it certainly suggests that its lack is an important factor. Zinc, amongst all the many other things, is important for brain development in the growing foetus. If there is a zinc deprivation in pregnancy there can be a defect of some sort in the offspring. Dyslexia does tend to run in families.

Autism

Doctors specializing in nutritional medicine, such as Dr Carl Pfeiffer, believe that autism is an environmental disorder. Autistic children have been found to have high copper and high lead levels. They are, in effect, suffering from heavy metal poisoning.

In the USA Dr Pfeiffer has been treating autistic children with the de-toxifying nutrients, specifically zinc and manganese and vitamin C together with vitamin B_6. According to Dr Pfeiffer, every autistic child he has treated in this way has improved. The observations of Dr Pfeiffer have been confirmed by Allan Cott and Catherine Spears, child neurologists in New York.

However, the nutritional approach is not the only effective one.

Specialist doctors are sometimes blinkered to approaches other than their own, and indeed often make fun of other disciplines. But as far as autism is concerned the approach involving 'holding sessions' should be considered too. In New York, Martha Welsh has achieved successes with autistic children with such 'holding sessions'. This means long, direct, skin-to-skin contact sessions between mother and child.

These two approaches could be complementary. In the holding sessions the child feels secure. So the level of the stress hormone cortisol, goes down. This then lowers the need for zinc and its co-workers. With the nutritional approach, the zinc and other nutrients are increased and adapt to specific hormonal balances.

Learning Difficulties and Delinquency

There is much in common between hyperactivity in children, autism, learning difficulties and delinquency. Learning problems, erratic and disruptive behaviour, inattentiveness and poor concentration are considered by some to be the symptoms of hyperactivity in an older child. Such problems may continue later on to become delinquency.

The elemental picture for all these conditions is one of heavy metal poisoning, particularly lead, and low levels of essential nutrients, including zinc. A mineral profile of a group of boys who were disruptive and violent in school showed them to be low in zinc, calcium, and manganese and high in cadmium, lead and iron.

The nutritional approach is the same as for the other conditions. It aims both to de-toxify the body of poisonous heavy metals, and raise the level of essential nutrients. So, once again, zinc is prescribed together with vitamin C, the B vitamins, vitamin D, E, calcium, magnesium, manganese, chromium, selenium, cobalt and essential fatty acids.

8

Zinc and Skin

The story of zinc and skin begins with pigs. In the middle 1950s vets discovered that zinc could cure a pig disease called parakeratose, a severe skin disease which also had symptoms of growth difficulties, digestive problems, loss of appetite and loss of weight. In the worst cases the pigs died. The illness only affected pigs who were on dry supplements of vegetable protein (peanuts, cottonseed and soya). Those that ate clover or alfalfa were unaffected. So a dietary cause was immediately suspected. Vitamins, minerals, amino-acids and antibiotics were all tried, and it was discovered that zinc carbonate had a spectacular effect, and that calcium and phosphorus made the illness worse. There was no doubt that the cause of this pig disease was too little zinc.

It was the same story with a skin disease in calves which is similar to eczema in humans. In 1975 *The Veterinary Journal of New Zealand* published the results of a wide-scale study of zinc treatment for eczema on the faces of calves. The study involved 150 calves from three different farms, all of which had facial eczema. One group of calves drank water to which had been added 6g of zinc sulphate per 100 litres, and the other group drank water to which no zinc had been added. The results were spectacular from the very start. Not only did the zinc make the skin lesions clear up, but it also had a dramatic effect on their weight-loss, their appetite and even their mortality. From these successes with animals, it was just a short leap to similar successes with zinc in skin conditions in humans.

In fact, zinc has been well-known to dermatologists for a long time. Zinc salts in solution, such as zinc chloride or zinc sulphate, have been used locally as light antiseptics for some skin conditions. And there has also been a variety of zinc powders, zinc ointments, and creams of zinc oxide which have been used for eczema, impetigo, ringworm, varicose ulcers and psoriasis. And for generations, mothers have been buying jars of zinc and castor oil cream from their local chemist to use as a protection or treatment against nappy rash on their babies' bottoms. None of this is new, but what is new is the use of zinc in dermatology for specific conditions. Acne is one of them.

Acne

There are countless medical publications which confirm the effectiveness of treating acne with zinc. They also state that when there is acne, there is usually a zinc deficiency at the same time. The most conclusive study was conducted by a Swedish group who compared the effects of zinc on its own, with vitamin A on its own, and with zinc and vitamin A together. The zinc was the most efficient.

Interestingly, acne is particularly common in adolescent boys. Puberty is the time when the prostate, the seminal vessels and the testicles are all growing rapidly. This calls for a sudden increase in zinc that in many cases is not being met.

There may be another reason, too, why adolescent boys are short of zinc and that reason is masturbation. It has been claimed that each ejaculation corresponds to a loss of 1mg of zinc. Without any moral overtones, it might be necessary to reconsider what medicine used to say about masturbation in the days when they thought it was a debilitating practice which lead to fatigue, loss of memory, weight loss and mental disturbances. In our more enlightened times masturbation is considered as a normal stage in sexual life and even has a therapeutic value. Nonetheless, one has to ask whether there might be a link between acne in adolescent boys and the frequent practice of masturbation.

Eczema

There is a promising future for zinc and its co-factors in the treatment of eczema. (See 'Allergic Conditions' in Chapter 7.)

There are basically two types of eczema; contact eczema and atopic eczema. The one which zinc may help is atopic eczema. This is an allergic disease which comes under the same heading as asthma or hay fever. Atopic eczema can appear as early as three to six months of age. When this happens there are usually other allergic illnesses in the family. The best way to reduce the chances of a child getting atopic eczema when the family is 'atopic' is to breastfeed exclusively for as long as possible. One has to be suspicious of even one little bottle of artificial milk given to a baby in the first days of its life, before the flow of breast milk has become established. When severe eczema begins in infancy there is unfortunately every chance that it will last a lifetime, although there are many exceptions to this, and there are also cases where eczema suddenly appears and disappears at any time of life.

There are really no totally satisfactory treatments for eczema. As it can last a lifetime, the important thing is to avoid using the kind of drugs which only have short-term effects, especially cortisone creams and ointments. Although they do calm the inflammation, they can actually encourage infection of the lesions. Cortisone creams and ointments are absorbed by the skin and can have side-effects. This means that anyone suffering from eczema should pay particular attention to the details of their daily life, such as what their clothes are made of, their lifestyle and their diet.

More and more nutritionists agree that the emphasis should be on a diet rich in essential fatty acids and zinc and its co-factors. There has been some success reported using zinc supplements of 50mg three times a day, together with 100mg vitamin C and 500mg evening primrose oil (3×3 times a day). It is too early to say whether this amounts to a new treatment, but even before firm proof, it would be a wise course of action to take.

Psoriasis

On the other hand, there is a skin disease for which the initial hopes of improvement by zinc have been disappointing. This is psoriasis, a skin disease whose characteristics are itchy red plaques, mostly on the scalp, back and elbows.

Psoriasis is not peculiar to our civilization in the same way the allergic diseases, cancer, depression, or circulatory diseases are. It might have been around since ancient times. Possibily the Hebrew word 'tsara'ath', sometimes translated as leprosy, in fact meant psoriasis.

Some dermatologists hoped that since psoriasis looked similar to parakeratose in pigs, zinc might do the trick. In 1969 a group of patients in Michigan were given 220mg of zinc sulphate a day, but they did no better than the control group who were given a placebo. It is now believed that there is nothing wrong with the absorption or metabolism of zinc in patients with psoriasis.

However, these observations do not exclude the possibility that high doses of zinc, taken with essential fatty acids and vitamins C and B_6 continuously and indefinitely can improve psoriasis. The Michigan study used zinc on its own, and only for two months. However, there are other studies in progress, and we will have to wait to see what they come up with.

There are still many unknown things about psoriasis. It seems to be associated with an insufficiency in the secretion of melatonin by the pineal gland, and a deep disturbance of the mobilization of arachidonic acid, the precursor of prostaglandins 2. This suggests that there may well be a specific imbalance between different prostaglandins, though genetic factors probably are involved in psoriasis as well.

Wound Healing

It is early days still on the subject of how zinc and its co-factors might help in wound healing. It is also possible that before too long zinc will be used in common childhood illnesses such as chicken pox and measles to help the skin heal quickly.

9
Colds and Zinc

Zinc as an effective treatment for the common cold is very new. A double-blind, placebo-controlled trial in Texas in 1983 proved that sucking zinc lozenges (23mg zinc gluconate) shortened the length of a cold by about seven days.

In the Texas trial, one group of 37 patients was given a 23mg zinc lozenge to suck every wakeful two hours, after an initial double dose. The control group was given a placebo of calcium lactate. After seven days, in 86% of the zinc-treated patients the cold had gone, compared with only 46% in the placebo group.

The way that these researchers hit upon zinc for colds is interesting, and was quite unexpected. They call it serendipity. One of the doctors, George A. Eby, observed a three-year-old girl having chemotherapy for leukaemia. She was also being given zinc in an effort to improve her zinc status and to stimulate the responsiveness of her T cells. This child suffered from frequent and severe colds both before and after her diagnosis of leukaemia.

The little girl refused to swallow one 50mg zinc tablet given to her by the doctors. She sucked it instead. And what the doctors noticed was that her cold disappeared without further treatment. Just in case this was sheer fluke, the doctors tried giving this child — and others — zinc lozenges to suck at each cold. It worked again and again, not just for the little girl in question but for the other children too, and adults as well.

In the Texas trial, which took place in collaboration with the local media, subjects with colds volunteered themselves. They recorded on a report form the presence and severity of ten common cold symptoms: headache; fever; muscle pain; sneezing; nasal drainage; nasal obstruction; sore throat; scratchy throat; cough and hoarseness. These symptoms were scored as being severe, moderate, minor, or absent. The subjects were also asked to record side-effects.

The researchers noted that zinc helped from the very start. In the zinc-treated group many lost their symptoms within hours (11% within 12 hours and 22% within 24 hours), whereas none of the placebo group lost their symptoms so fast. At the end of the seven-day experiment 86% of the zinc-treated group reported all their cold symptoms gone, compared with only 46% of the placebo subjects.

Side-Effects

Quite a few people (23%) dropped out of the zinc-treated group, complaining about the unpleasant taste, distortion of taste and mouth irritation. A few people reported vomiting and nausea, but this seems to have been preventable by eating and drinking before taking the tablets.

How Does Zinc Work in Colds?

The Texas doctors aren't exactly sure how zinc relieves colds, but they have put forward some hypotheses. They say that zinc probably works by inhibiting viral polypeptide cleavage, although they have no proof of this. Another possibility is that zinc minimizes histamine release from mast cells and basophils at an anti-viral concentration. Another possibility is the immunoregulation of T-cell lymphocytes, or the prevention of excessive immunosuppressive T-cell production by means of inhibition of histamine release. Zinc treatment may also mimic or increase a previously unrecognized anti-viral function of mast cells and basophils.

Zinc Works Best at the First Signs of a Cold

One thing which emerged from the Texas study was that zinc works best on early symptoms of a cold rather than on a full-blown cold. The doctors observed that incipient colds of only a few hours old often seemed to abort within several hours, although they admit this was not put to any scientific test.

Which Zinc Compound Works Best?

The Texas researchers used unflavoured zinc gluconate tablets, but they are the first to admit that this could be improved upon, as they are rather unpleasant to taste. They tried zinc orotate and found it was substantially less effective. Zinc sulphate and zinc chloride were not tested due to reports of very painful and caustic effects on mucous membranes.

Apart from lozenges to suck, they tried other methods, but none worked so well. Swallowing zinc tablets did not seem to work in the same way as sucking them. Nasal sprays did work but needed to be administered too frequently to be practical (every 10 to 15 minutes). They also caused some discomfort.

Since the trials, zinc lozenges have come on the market as a treatment for colds. They are zinc gluconate 23mg, but the metallic zinc taste is disguised with peppermint flavour and they are nice to suck. These products are easy to find in chemists shops throughout the UK.

Dose

The researchers feared that any anti-viral effect of zinc could be reversible. So they felt it was important to administer lozenges frequently, including the first six hours after all the cold symptoms had gone away. Adults were given 23mg zinc gluconate every two hours while awake. The first dose was double this amount. The maximum was twelve tablets a day; nine for youths. The treatment lasted only seven days. Children under 60lbs (27kg) received half a tablet every two hours while awake, not exceeding six tablets a day.

The Texas researchers, although very happy with their results, say that further studies are needed to confirm what they found.

10

Herpes

A rapist can be sentenced to an additional five years in prison if he gives herpes to his victim, a California court ruled recently. This shows the seriousness with which herpes is viewed. Herpes is an important issue of public health. As a sexually transmitted disease it is of concern during pregnancy. It can present life-threatening risks for a baby. There is also a relationship between herpes and cancer of the cervix, and cancer of the uterus.

The incidence of genital herpes has increased considerably in the last two decades. There are some 500,000 new cases of herpes a year in the USA, and medical consultations for herpes increased tenfold between 1960 and 1979. Today, genital herpes is more frequent than syphilis and gonorrhoea, at least in some social classes.

The first attack can be dramatic, with fever, general malaise, genital pain, vaginal discharge, which can be bloody, and pain on urinating. In a typical case there are small vesicles, or superficial ulceration, of the genital organs, with enlarged glands in the groin. This first attack is normally over in one to three weeks. Usually there are relapses. Indeed, the condition is characterized by a series of recurrences. These flare-ups are in general less dramatic, less painful and shorter — lasting only ten days or so.

As yet there is no satisfactory treatment for genital herpes, although anti-viral drugs such as vidarabine and acyclovar are commonly used. Acyclovar can shorten a relapse but cannot reduce the frequency of relapses and it cannot get to the reserves of the virus in the ganglions.

Zinc in the Treatment of Herpes

Zinc shows promise in the treatment of herpes. It has been used both on the sores on the skin, and taken by mouth to work nutritionally. Herpes is incurable, but the aim of any treatment is to try to prolong remissions and delay relapses. The first thing to do is to try to understand the factors which trigger relapses. Any situation which depresses the immune system encourages recurrences. When immuno-suppressive drugs are used these recurrences can be very serious. The chances of a relapse can be increased at the start of menstruation, during a fever, from exposure to sunlight, from certain emotions and from surgery.

In addition, laboratory studies have shown that a high level of prostaglandins 2 (E_2) suppresses the response of lymphocytes to the herpes virus, and this encourages relapses, too. Indeed, all the circumstances which encourage relapses go with an imbalance between the different series of prostaglandins, and probably an imbalance which tips prostaglandins 2 too high.

The use of zinc and its co-factors makes sense theoretically. This is because they are necessary for the production of prostaglandins 1, and for maintaining a good balance between the different series of prostaglandins. It is too early to make any claims for this yet, as time is needed to properly evaluate this regimen. Even so, it would be wise to avoid toxic drugs, and do everything to reinforce the immune system by simple and safe means, as a first resort.

Zinc for Herpes Sores on the Skin

There have been several successful trials using local treatments for herpes, starting in 1975 with the use of zinc sulphate solutions for herpetic lesions. It is known that a zinc ion can inhibit the replication of the herpes simplex virus.

A Swedish dermatologist by the name of Isser Brody has done some very successful work on herpes of the mouth, using zinc sulphate solutions. Herpes of the mouth, otherwise known as cold sores, are due to the herpes simplex virus type 1. Isser Brody found out which solutions of zinc sulphate worked best for cold sores. He showed that the zinc sulphate solutions usually used in dermatology are too strong (0.2 to 1%) and that in cold sores on the mouth such strong solutions could cause irritation, mouth dryness and nausea. He found that the best concentration on the skin was 0.025-0.5%, and the best concentration for use on the mucous membrane on the mouth should not be stronger than 0.01-0.025%. He used a gauze compress soaked in a lukewarm zinc sulphate solution. His method was to keep them on the lesions for about ten minutes during the acute periods; once a day until the sores disappeared. After that, he recommended a maintenance treatment of once a week for the first month, and then twice a month.

Although Isser Brody's work involved the herpes simplex virus 1, the dividing line between the type 1 and the type 2 virus is rather vague. So it would not be a long shot to use the same treatment for the skin lesions of genital herpes. It might be a way of limiting the spread of lesions. The first results using zinc sulphate solutions look promising.

Genital Herpes, Pregnancy and Childbirth

In the absence of other treatments, it would be safe to use zinc sulphate solutions on genital herpes in a pregnant woman. Often, a selective caesarian is planned for a woman with recurrent herpes, even without being able to know in advance whether or not the lesions will be active at the time of the birth.

I know several women who refused to have a caesarian. At the time of childbirth none of these women had visible lesions. In cases like these it is especially important to avoid artificial rupture of the membranes, and even to avoid any kind of vaginal examination.

In cases such as this, the serum of the baby contains the same level of anti-herpetic antibodies as the serum of the mother, because they cross the placenta. These antibodies can still be found after the age of six months. A study demonstrated that, if the newborn baby is infected, the degree of infection depends on the level of antibodies.

A planned caesarian in cases where the pregnant woman has genital herpes is debatable; it is not a way to absolutely prevent the newborn baby from being affected. Some babies are infected in the womb during the pregnancy.

Of course, everything should be done to limit the spread of herpes. But at the same time one needs to hold on to an objective appreciation of the true risks, and not resort to panic measures. The risk of death to the newborn baby is low compared to the huge frequency of the disease in western countries. Most pregnant women who have recurrent herpes do not have lesions at the time of the delivery — perhaps because a spontaneous delivery means a hormonal balance which prevents a relapse. Also, even when the baby must go through an infected genital canal to be born, it still has a 50% chance of not getting a disseminated infection. Disseminated infection is in itself compatible with a survival rate of around 50%. Disseminated infection involves the central nervous system, the conjunctiva, the meninges and the skin.

In 1980, the American Academy of Pediatrics recommended a weekly systematic research of the virus on the cervix in the last weeks of pregnancy in all those pregnant women who had a history of herpes. Only those women with two consecutive negative tests would be allowed to give birth by the vaginal route. The others would be selected for caesarian deliveries.

It has been calculated that this system would avoid no more than 30 cases of newborn babies with herpes a year for the whole of the USA, at a cost of $1.8m for each avoided case, and 3.3 maternal deaths arising from the greater number of complications associated with a higher number of caesarians.

In conclusion, zinc used both as a solution directly on the skin, and nutritionally with its co-workers to boost the immune system, could be tried first in cases of genital herpes, and herpes of the mouth.

11

Anorexia Nervosa

Anorexia nervosa is an increasingly common disease of our civilization, and one of the most mysterious. Yet it holds several clues about the metabolism of zinc.

The disease is centuries old, but it is certainly on the increase today. In 1689 it was described by Richard Merton as 'nervous consumption'. He wrote that a female patient suffering from this condition was 'only a skeleton clad in skin'. But while in the past anorexia nervosa was one of those diseases you read about in textbooks but were never likely to meet, today everyone knows first-hand about these adolescent girls who suddenly refuse to eat.

Typically, these girls belong to small families with a high standard of living. Such families are considered to be happy, stable and success-orientated. Anorexia seems to be an illness which affects the nuclear family. Such a soil is fertile for anorexia when the parents are dedicated and ambitious, with a tendency to overestimate their child. There is often an obese person in the family circle.

Anorexia usually starts in adolescence, and affects ten times more women than men. The girl's perception of her own body becomes distorted. The illness often starts with an event which touches on the girl's sexuality, such as a film or a course on sex education. The girl feels unhappy with the way she is; her figure in particular.

This dissatisfaction with her body image is reinforced by advertisements in the media which always project women as slim and beautiful. But even when an anorexic girl gets very slim, by any objective standards, she may still look at herself in the mirror and think she looks fat. Following the first crisis the anorexic girl's periods often stop altogether. Her decision to slim involves not only eating less, but often the use of laxatives or induced vomiting, or intense sporting activity such as long runs or swims.

The disease has really caught hold when the girl is no longer in control of her weight loss; when she has lost her sense of taste, and lost all urge to eat. It is a vicious circle. Very recently it was found that if these girls agreed to take a zinc supplement it broke the vicious circle, and some spectacular cures have been reported.

Note: Because both anorexia nervosa and bulimia respond in a similar way to zinc, some nutritionists make a link between them.

Anorexia and Zinc

Some people think that anorexia is due to a lack of zinc; but this may be too simplistic, although once the disease has taken hold the ability to absorb zinc from the gut is very much lowered.

Certainly, anorexia *becomes* a condition of zinc deficiency simply because the girl is eating very little food. Our opinion is that a lack of zinc is not a cause of anorexia. If that were the case, why is anorexia hardly ever found in families in lower socio-economic groups where the diet tends to be poor in protein and zinc and high in saturated fats and refined sugar?

There is another possible explanation. This hypothesis takes account of some factors which are often overlooked. Girls who suffer from anorexia rarely get colds and seem to escape 'flu epidemics. Studies have shown that the cell-mediated immunity of anorexics is perfectly intact. Here is the essential difference between anorexia and situations of food deprivation which are generally accompanied by a depression of the immune system.

In anorexia, the girl chooses not to eat out of her own free will — it is voluntary behaviour. Whereas in the case of most other situations of food deprivation, a person can do nothing about it but submit passively. In circumstances of helplessness like this, higher amounts of cortisol are secreted and this high level of cortisol depresses the functions of the thymus, thus depressing the immune system. But, with the anorexic, it is her voluntary behaviour which keeps her immune system intact. A girl who struggles hard to slim down, who freely decides to stick to a diet, is not in a situation where a high level of cortisol is secreted. She may indeed be unhappy about her body image, but she does not show the classic signs of depression.

As far as zinc is concerned, the anorexic girl — who has an increased need for zinc during adolescence anyway — reserves what zinc she has for vital functions. The priority is the immune system, which is kept in good working order. So the first signs of any shortage of zinc do not show up in the immune system. The first signs of zinc deficiency will be a loss of taste and smell. Once that happens, food loses its attraction. It also seems that a change in the intestinal mucosa makes it unable to absorb zinc.

This is how the vicious circle takes hold — a vicious circle which can be broken by taking zinc supplements. If the anorexic girl is compliant in taking enough zinc, her interest in food will come back and her intestinal mucosa will recover its capacity to absorb zinc.

It is important to state yet again that the girls who are most likely to get anorexia nervosa usually belong to the higher socio-economic groups. So they are very representative of western society with a high standard of living. Their way of life up until the time they get anorexia might make them especially vulnerable to a lack of zinc. This ironic situation needs to be explained.

These girls have been accustomed since infancy to a varied, high quality diet rich in bio-available zinc. What happens when they suddenly starve themselves is their bodies cannot cope with this sudden and drastic drop in zinc. They have become dependent on high levels of zinc, and cannot adapt to situations where it is no longer present.

Our interpretation of anorexia nervosa shows that it is quite different from depressive illnesses whose symptoms are inactivity, resignation, sadness and letting events take over. It is also different from most other situations of food deprivation which are usually not chosen out of free will but are situations people can do nothing about.

12

Depression

Zinc supplements can help depression. In depressed people there is a high level of cortisol, and cortisol tends to block the metabolism of unsaturated fatty acids and the synthesis of prostaglandins.

The 'Nouvelle Medicine' approach would be to increase your intake of zinc, vitamin C, vitamin B_6, the other B vitamins and essential fatty acids. In certain respects, veterinary medicine is more advanced than human medicine when it comes to treating animals with a 'Nouvelle Medicine' approach. Here is one story to illustrate that.

Like all livestock breeders, Mrs Gladys Reid, a farmer in New Zealand, knew that if you separated newborn calves from their mothers it is traumatic for them and badly affects their health. Such calves become depressed and refuse to eat. Their tails get dirty because they can't be bothered to raise them when they defecate.

This farmer noticed that when she added zinc sulphate to the feed in their troughs, it completely transformed the calves' behaviour. The day after they had eaten the feed containing zinc the calves frolicked in the fields, grazed peacefully and raised their tails to defecate. Mrs Reid noticed that by adding zinc to the calves' feed they stayed healthy throughout the weaning period.

Until now it was impossible to give these rural observations the true importance they deserve. A calf separated from its mother is in a hopeless situation. He can do nothing but submit. This is what Henri Laborit meant by 'inhibition of action'. Others prefer to call it helplessness. This depression, this submissive behaviour, is accompanied by a high secretion of cortisol and a diminished need to struggle for survival.

It is known that the hormone cortisol blocks some important metabolic pathways, especially the ones which lead to the synthesis of prostaglandins. If the organism gets used to secreting a high level of cortisol all the time it is virtually asking for physiological suicide — it makes no difference what the symptoms are, or how you label the disease.

Under circumstances such as these the immune system is depressed; the level of cholesterol is raised; the arteries thicken; the small blood vessels contract; the skin worsens and opens the way for infections; all the tissues degenerate, and so do the joints.

When a calf is given zinc supplements, it counteracts cortisol, encouraging the chemical reactions which were blocked by cortisol. The calf loses his attitude of resignation, he no longer behaves in a submissive way with its cascade of consequences, including refusing to eat. The vicious circle is broken. It is interesting to note that the farmer did not use an anti-depressive drug. Instead, she looked for something which would satisfy the basic needs of the calves. It would be worthwhile telling this story of the New Zealand calves to all young medical students, both now and in the future, while they are at an age when their ideas about health, disease and the doctor's role are still being formed.

Such a story voices the question of the millions of babies all over the world who are separated from their mothers in hospitals which purport to be primarily concerned with caring for their health. The question has to be asked whether so many babies really need to be isolated in a glass box called an incubator, rather than have direct skin-to-skin contact with their mother. In Bogotà, the capital of Colombia, it is possible for a high percentage of babies who weigh less than 1 kilo at birth to survive. There, they use what is known as the 'kangaroo' method which means keeping the low birth-weight babies against their mothers breasts day and night, held securely and kept very warm.

Post-Natal Depression

Some doctors and biochemists now believe that post-natal depression is a condition of zinc deficiency which can be cured almost magically by giving zinc supplements. Perhaps the best source of zinc for new mothers is the placenta. Some mothers already follow the example of animals and eat some of their own placenta to get a good supply of minerals. An alternative would be for manufacturers to make freeze-dried placenta tablets. In the meantime, conventional zinc supplements would do. The zinc level in the mother-to-be drops in the last two to three days of pregnancy, when zinc is transferred to the baby. So far, the few people who have been suggesting zinc for post-natal depression report very good results.

Seasonal Depression

Zinc supplements might be especially useful in seasonal depression. This is when the symptoms appear at the end of autumn and disappear when spring arrives. Seasonal depression might be interpreted as an inability to adapt to darkness. Too low a level of melatonin from the pineal gland is part of the explanation for this. Melatonin has the effect of putting a brake on the adrenal gland, and its action is often in opposition to cortisol. Exposure to artificial bright lights before daybreak and after nightfall over a long period of time is one way of reducing the effects of seasonal depression.

Note
Although zinc and its co-workers are good for depression, paradoxically the depression can worsen at the start of the zinc treatment. This happens when copper is being freed from certain tissues.

Rheumatoid Arthritis and Schizophrenia: Models for a 'Nouvelle Medicine'

Rheumatoid Arthritis

Classifying diseases gets more and more difficult. Under what heading, for example, should one put that common type of rheumatism, rheumatoid arthritis? It would be possible, of course, to classify rheumatoid arthritis as a rheumatic disease, like all joint and muscle pains which are not directly connected with either an infection or a wound. It would also be possible, though, to classify rheumatoid arthritis as an inflammatory disease. These days, rheumatoid arthritis tends to be considered as an illness involving the immune system — an auto-immune disease. Perhaps a virus is involved, in which case it would be classified as a viral disease.

But no matter how you classify it, there are some things about rheumatoid arthritis which are certain. It is a chronic disease. One person in twenty will get this disease at some time in their lives if they live in the western world. Most of the symptoms are due to inflammation of the fibrous tissues surrounding the joints. Every joint can be affected, but the most common are the knuckles and the wrists. In a typical case, there is a small inflamed nodule just under the skin. In some people the disease starts in childhood or adolescence and can go on all their lives. The illness can turn people into invalids, with terribly stiff joints (especially first thing in the morning), swellings and deformed limbs.

One detailed study on rheumatoid arthritis looked at 88 children with juvenile arthritis. They found that in many cases the disease was preceded by some emotional trauma, such as family bereavement, divorce of the parents, or being adopted. Traumas such as these can have a powerful effect on the immune system.

Anti-Inflammatory Drugs

In the last few decades the usual treatments for rheumatoid arthritis have come from the cul-de-sac of conventional medicine. Most of these treatments have been used throughout the world on a massive scale, but only their short-term benefits have been considered. Their long-term side-effects, which can be terrible, have not been taken into account. It would be hard to justify them for a disease which is, after all, not life-threatening.

The drug cortisone, and other drugs of the same group (the corticosteroids) were first used for rheumatoid arthritis. Their effects on the immune system, on the bones, on the blood-pressure and on behaviour were not considered. Later, the non-steroidal anti-inflammatory drugs came along (NSAIDs); drugs such as butazolidine, tanderil and indocid. They were used by millions of people, until the time when they had to be completely withdrawn from the market, except for very special cases. This happened when their side-effects, sometimes fatal, came to light and it was realized that their risks outweighed their benefits.

The dangers of aspirin in the treatment of chronic diseases have also been underestimated. There is a real risk of stomach ulcers; of haemorrhaging, especially in the digestive tract; there can be subtle damage to the ear; and problems for people with allergies. All this was unknown for a long time. But nowadays it is possible to see why anti-inflammatory drugs can have dangerous side-effects in the long term.

The priority of the anti-inflammatory drugs is to block the route to prostaglandins 2 (thromboxane A2 in particular). These are the prostaglandins which reinforce the inflammatory processes. By blocking these prostaglandins, these drugs are able to bring immediate relief and do alleviate the symptoms. But this disguises the fact that these drugs in fact make the illness worse. This is because they not only block the route to prostaglandins 2, but also limit the access to prostaglandins 1 (and to prostacycline).

Prostaglandins 1 are themselves anti-inflammatory, and are indispensable for the immune system to work well. A good balance between the different types of prostaglandins is itself a condition of good health. It seems that in most of the diseases of civilization, there is a tendency towards a deficit of prostaglandins 1 (and perhaps prostaglandins 3 as well) and towards a relative excess of prostaglandins 2. Once you realize this, it is easy to understand how the anti-inflammatory drugs can have such a wide range of bad side-effects.

The plug which blocks the route to prostaglandins 2 also reduces the passage towards prostaglandins 1 at the same time. This is how drugs like corticosteroids, aspirin, and anti-inflammatory drugs work.

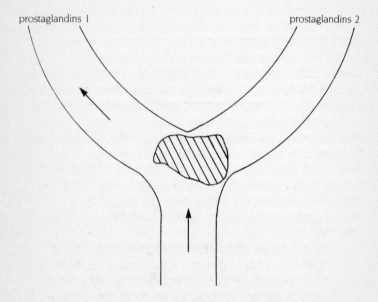

Figure 4. Conventional medicine: how anti-inflammatory drugs work

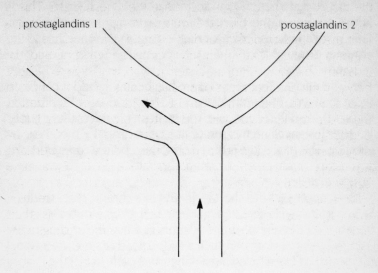

Figure 5. 'Nouvelle Medicine'

Every means possible is used to increase the route towards prostaglandins 1. This includes zinc, vitamin C, vitamin B_6, unsaturated fatty acids including GLA, positive emotions.

Other Drugs

Some people have put forward the view that the route towards prostaglandins 1 might be made even wider by using drugs which stimulate the manufacture of prostaglandins 1. This is how the drug colchicine works, which has a well-established reputation in the treatment of gout. Chloroquine, well known for the prevention and treatment of malaria, works in the same way. Penicillin too has been used like this.

However, prudence needs to be exercised when prescribing drugs for a chronic disease. The drugs mentioned above might have a low toxicity, but this is not the case for some other drugs being prescribed for rheumatoid arthritis in which a high toxicity is obvious. Some of these drugs have long-term irreversible effects. Take, for example, the trials for methotrexate which belongs to the group of drugs which kill cells by blocking the action of essential enzymes.

In some instances methotrexate has been injected locally into the joints, with immediate effects which have been interpreted differently by different people. This carries a big risk of liver toxicity. In other instances methotrexate has been given by mouth or by injection. This procedure is based on some reported cases of instant success in certain types of rheumatism such as Reiter's syndrome or polymyositis.

These successes are short term. But in a chronic disease which is not in itself life-threatening their side-effects outweigh their benefits, so the use of drugs like this is a matter for debate. By using aggressive drugs on such a widespread scale, conventional medicine has been following a dangerous path. In fact the history of the treatment of rheumatoid arthritis illustrates perfectly the two attitudes to medicine — attitudes which are radically opposed to each other and hard to reconcile. But surely it is time now to call a halt to past errors and find a new approach — a 'Nouvelle Medicine'.

'Nouvelle Medicine' and Zinc

The approach of 'Nouvelle Medicine' is radically different from the orthodox approach. It is less simplistic; it is in less of a hurry to suppress symptoms; it is more concerned with maintaining good health. Instead of trying to block the synthesis of prostaglandins 2, its aim is to open the route to prostaglandins 1 as widely as possible. Zinc is very important to this new approach. The beneficial effects of zinc for people with rheumatism have been reported in the most orthodox medical literature. Since the early 1970s zinc has been used extensively at the Brain Bio Center in New Jersey. Of course, zinc's action is reinforced by other elements which work in the same way, especially vitamin C and vitamin B_6, and essential fatty acids such as evening primrose oil. This therapy involves cutting back on animal fats, refined oils and sugar. On the subject of sugar, new research has shown that a rapid increase in the blood sugar level increases sensitivity to pain. This is particularly relevant to people suffering from rheumatoid arthritis.

In such a strategy, zinc might have several different modes of action. Not only does zinc favour the synthesis of the anti-inflammatory prostaglandins and stimulate the thymus and the immune system, but it also tends to rid the body of excessive amounts of copper and iron in diseased joints.

This nutritional approach cannot be described as a treatment in the proper sense of the word. You cannot expect instant spectacular results, and instead have to be patient to reap the benefits.

It is clear that for the time being conventional medicine is not ready for such a radical change of direction. Thinking still tends to be that any nutritional approach, including the use of zinc, does not deserve to be taken seriously. In reviewing a recent book about rheumatoid arthritis a distinguished rheumatologist wrote: 'It was difficult to find any ommission, especially after reading an entire chapter on remedies of unlikely benefit which covers such diverse therapies as zinc, acupuncture, cocaine and prayer, all neatly referenced!' His exclamation mark underlines the huge gap between the two types of medicine.

Schizophrenia

Schizophrenia has quite a lot in common with rheumatoid arthritis, although their similarities may not be obvious. A little known fact is that these two illnesses exclude each other — people with rheumatoid arthritis are protected against schizophrenia and vice versa. The common factor between both diseases seems to be an imbalance between different prostaglandins. It is possible that a lack of prostaglandins 1 is one of the keys to schizophrenia. This particular hypothesis is the only way to make a link between all the various treatments and observations to do with schizophrenia.

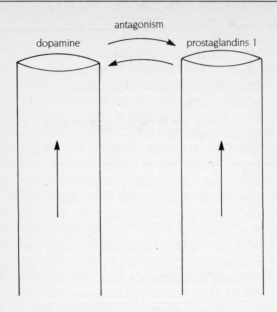

Figure 6. The route towards dopamine and prostaglandins 1

For example, it is known that fever, and epileptic fits, both of which stimulate the formation of prostaglandins 1, bring about remissions in schizophrenics. Most anti-schizophrenic drugs stimulate the secretion of the hormone prolactin, a hormone which encourages the synthesis of prostaglandins 1. At the same time most of these drugs block the receptors to a brain messenger called dopamine. Conversely, drugs which exaggerate the secretion of dopamine, such as amphetamines and cocaine, can elicit the kind of behaviour one associates with schizophrenia. Also, the prostaglandins and dopamine are antagonistic.

Just as conventional medicine attempts to block the synthesis of prostaglandins 2 in the case of rheumatoid arthritis, so does it try and block dopamine in schizophrenia. In both cases, the approach is to block some metabolic pathways which are over-active.

This is of course radically different from the approach of 'Nouvelle Medicine,' which first tries to build up those physiological processes which might be deficient. Its first aim is to help the synthesis and the actions of prostaglandins 1, and prostacycline. The two opposing medical viewpoints are illustrated in Figures 7 and 8.

Zinc and Schizophrenia

Zinc and its co-factors help by enlarging the route towards prostaglandins 1. One particularly spectacular result was reported using zinc with vitamin B_6. Others used zinc with GLA in evening primrose oil. Others tried penicillin, which also works by aiding the synthesis of prostaglandins 1.

Giving schizophrenics zinc and its co-factors has much to

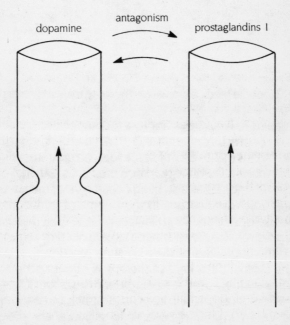

Figure 7. Conventional medicine reduces the routes towards dopamine

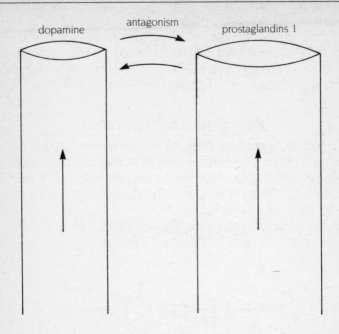

Figure 8. 'Nouvelle Medicine' enlarges the route towards prostaglandins 1

recommend it. Firstly, this approach is supported by all existing theories about schizophrenia and there have been some reported successes. Zinc makes a lot of sense for schizophrenics since many schizophrenics have white marks on their nails — the tell-tale signs of zinc deficiency. It has also been observed that there are specific proteins which bind to zinc in the plasma of schizophrenics.

An intake of zinc and its co-factors has the added advantage of working well on the allergies often experienced by schizophrenics and on the anomalies of their immune functions.

At the moment this kind of therapy is rare for schizophrenics. Much more widely used are neuroleptic drugs, or ECT treatment. Neuroleptic drugs can help in an acute attack, but they are usually ineffective when the patient is in a more chronic state of schizophrenia, as if cut off from normal life. They have no effect on his behaviour or his emotional responses.

There would be nothing to lose and everything to gain from trying zinc and its co-factors first.

Dr Carl Pfeiffer of the Brain Bio Center in New Jersey has been using zinc plus vitamin B_6, together with some other nutrients, for all his schizophrenic patients with very dramatic results. He has found schizophrenics to be 'pyroluric', which means they were found to be losing zinc and B_6 in their urine.

14

Which Supplements of Zinc?

Probably the easiest way to take zinc is in the form of a commercial supplement and the choice of these is growing all the time. But there are certain things you need to know in order to buy wisely.

How Much Zinc Is Really in the Supplement?

Figures can be misleading. There is a difference between the quantity of zinc salts, and the amount of elemental zinc. For example, a product advertising itself as having Zinc Gluconate 23mg only has in fact 3mg of the metal zinc in each tablet. So read the label very carefully, especially the small print.

Zinc sulphate is probably the most widely used zinc salt. 100mg of zinc sulphate contains 22.7mg of metal. Many preparations contain 220mg of salt, which means about 50mg of the metal.

What's the Difference Between Zinc Sulphate, Zinc Orotate, Zinc Gluconate etc?

Zinc Sulphate

These are the cheapest and most commonly used zinc salts. It has been said that any pharmacist can make a solution of it, and it would only cost one penny to buy enough zinc sulphate to last a whole month! Unfortunately, commercial supplements of zinc sulphate cost considerably more than that. A supplementary dose would be 220mg a day, which supplies 50mg of elemental zinc. Zinc sulphate is tolerated better if it is taken with a meal.

Zinc Orotate

A synthetic derivative, combined with orotic acid. It is claimed by some to be better absorbed than zinc salts, although others disagree with this. It is also said to facilitate passage through the cell membranes. Zinc orotate was the choice of Dr Alec Forbes when he was at the Bristol Cancer Help Centre. It provides 17mg of zinc in 100mg. It is well tolerated. Orotic acid is still sometimes called vitamin B_{13} but, as large amounts of it are made by the body, it is no longer recognized by some as having the status of a vitamin.

Zinc Citrate

A less common supplement of zinc is zinc citrate. The advantage of zinc citrate is that it makes both the absorption of zinc and manganese easier. (One problem with zinc supplements is that as the zinc level goes up, the manganese level goes down. See page 101).

Zinc Gluconate

Zinc gluconate is used primarily for the treatment of the common cold. In some countries it is sold in the form of lozenges which contain 23mg zinc gluconate. Gluconate contains 13mg of zinc per 100mg. The dose for adults is to suck 2 lozenges to begin with, then one every two hours while awake, with a maximum of 10 tablets a day. The children's dose is half a lozenge every 2 hours, not exceeding 6 lozenges a day. Because the lozenge is sucked and not swallowed, it means that the zinc is being absorbed through the mouth and not through the gut.

Chelations of Zinc

Chelate means latch onto, or bind to something else. Zinc is normally absorbed by binding to proteins. Zinc amino-acid chelate provides

10mg zinc in 100mg. Based on animal and human studies, it is claimed to be more efficiently absorbed than other zinc supplements. The supplement dose is 150-200mg zinc chelate a day, which supplies 15-20mg of zinc.

Zinc and Vitamin B_6

Zinc is always absorbed and used better when it is together with vitamin B_6.

Can Zinc Be Toxic?

There is a very wide margin between dietary needs and toxic doses. Compared with other minerals, such as copper, selenium, lead, cadmium and mercury, zinc has virtually no toxicity. The rare cases of zinc toxification were from things like inhaling zinc fumes in smelting plants. Poisoning can sometimes happen from drinking acidic drinks which had been stored in a zinc-galvanized container. Pharmaceutically acceptable forms of zinc are generally regarded as non-cumulative and non-toxic. This would be at about 100-200mg a day. Most excess zinc is not absorbed and is excreted in the faeces. The Mineral Safety Index for zinc is very high: 33. This is the ratio between the minimum toxic dose (500mg) and the recommended daily intake. Even a case of extreme abuse of zinc gluconate, reported by some Texan doctors, left no lasting bad effects. In this case, the person took 10-20 times the above dose every two hours for months. This resulted in anaemia, neutropenia, very high alkaline phosphatase, a serum zinc concentration ten times higher than normal, and a serum copper concentration one tenth of normal. These abnormal findings were reversed with no apparent harm after the person stopped taking zinc and was given trace amounts of copper to compensate for the loss.

This case illustrates how habitual or long-term ingestion of high doses of zinc may be hazardous — not because zinc is toxic but because it creates imbalances with copper and other nutrients too. This cannot be justified for treating colds or for attempting to prevent them.

Does Zinc Have Side-Effects?

A very large dose of zinc sulphate could make you feel sick, and cause vomiting and diarrhoea. This would be if you took as much as half a gram to 2 grams.

The Risk of Creating a Mineral Imbalance

Somebody recently likened the minerals to the balls on a snooker table — if you hit one ball, all the other balls are affected. This book has been concentrating on zinc, but it is very important to take zinc in a balance with other minerals. It is now believed that zinc should ideally be taken with manganese. This is because as your zinc level goes up the manganese goes down. As manganese is vital for many functions a supplement of manganese should be taken at the same time as a zinc supplement. Dr Carl Pfeiffer believes that zinc and manganese should be taken in almost equal amounts. (15mg elemental zinc together with 10mg manganese.) Taking zinc in pharmacological doses without added manganese runs the risk of creating a manganese deficiency.

There are several examples in the past of one supplement creating imbalances of other important nutrients. For example, supplements of calcium or iron taken on their own during pregnancy, or supplements of vitamin D given to children. It would be a pity for zinc to fall into the same trap.

The study of zinc's actions in the body always brings us back to the concepts of balance, antagonism, complementarity and auto-regulation. Zinc should never be seen in isolation. It is part of a whole team. All nutrients are interdependent and all people are biochemically unique.

How Much Zinc Should You Take?

One person may need more zinc than another, so there is no universal answer, but having said that, it would be safe to take 15mg of elemental zinc twice a day, making a total of 30mg of supplemental zinc a day.

The one exception to this is in the case of epilepsy. In order to avoid the risk of a grand mal seizure, an epileptic should always start by taking vitamin B_6 and manganese *before* starting zinc.

The other thing to watch out for is falling into the trap of thinking that more means better. Some people who have had themselves tested for their mineral status and who have been found to be low in zinc have wrongly assumed that by taking very large supplements from the start, they will make up the shortfall of zinc faster. But in fact this does not seem to be the case at all. Dr Carl Pfeiffer has found that when somebody is severely zinc deficient, it is probably better to start them off on a relatively low dose and build them up gradually to a higher dose. The trouble with starting with a very high dose, is that you have to keep it up. Nobody yet knows exactly why this is.

What Else Should You Take With Zinc?

At the present time, it seems that zinc should ideally be taken with the following:

> Vitamin B_6 (50mg twice a day)
> Vitamin C (from 1 gram twice a day)
> Essential fatty acids (3×500mg evening primrose oil capsules twice a day)
> Manganese (10mg twice a day. This is more than you need but manganese is badly absorbed)
> Magnesium (10mg twice a day is ample)
> Nicotinic Acid (15mg twice a day)

It is now thought that molybdenum could usefully be added to this list. If you wanted to make sure you were including enough anti-oxidants, include:

> Vitamin E (natural not synthetic)
> Selenium
> Superoxide dismutase

Beware: Your Body Gets Used to High Doses of Zinc

As we mentioned opposite, the risk of starting supplements of zinc on a high dose is that your body comes to expect a high dose of zinc all the time. It becomes dependent on a high dose. Once you start doing this, you have to keep it up all the time, as a sudden drop would itself cause problems. As well as dependency, there is even a notion of addiction to particular catalysts.

We have seen that people who have been vegetarians since childhood seem to need less zinc than people who switched to vegetarianism once they were adults. These people, who had been eating animal proteins (rich in zinc) since childhood were dependent on that high level of zinc. So they need correspondingly more zinc when they stop eating the foods they had been used to. The same theory applies to anorexia nervosa.

There is one dramatic case of zinc deficiency in the medical literature which was thought by the researchers to be a case of addiction to zinc and other nutrients. The story is about a newborn baby girl, born normally at term weighing 3.2kg. Before long, the baby got sores on her skin and eyelids. She had diarrhoea; she was irritable, and generally unwell. Doctors thought of zinc deficiency, and indeed this was confirmed in the laboratory. The little girl made a spectacular recovery on zinc. The zinc treatment was tailed off later and then stopped completely.

Since birth, the baby had been fed on an artificial milk which contained a balanced amount of zinc and iron. The doctors came to the conclusion that the only possible explanation was that the mother had been taking various supplements during the last seven months of her pregnancy: zinc (20-40mg daily) together with different B and C vitamins. So this particular case of zinc deficiency could be interpreted as a sudden deprivation after a long period of relative abundance. Breastfeeding is probably the best way of avoiding this, as the mother is unlikely to change her dietary habits abruptly after the birth. Nevertheless, this case does have a serious lesson which people could learn from.

Other Supplements Containing Zinc

Spirulina

There are other ways of taking zinc apart from the simple zinc supplements. Spirulina is one of them. It is a microscopic blue algae, which might have first appeared on this earth as long as 3,000,000,000 years ago. The nutritional properties of spirulina were only discovered in 1963, by scientists working at the French Institute of Petrol.

Not only does spirulina contain an appreciable quantity of zinc (about 3mg per 100g), the zinc in spirulina is together with all its main co-factors, especially all the B vitamins, biotin, vitamin E, and magnesium. Above all, spirulina is an exceptional source of unsaturated fatty acids, not only linoleic acid (more than 10g per kg) but also GLA (about 10g per kg). What is more, spirulina is a good source of protein (70%). In fact it is the richest in protein of all natural sources. These proteins contain a large amount of an amino acid called phenylalamine, which acts directly on the regulatory centres of appetite. So spirulina is also good news as part of a slimming diet. The nutritional elements in spirulina are highly digestible because the membrane is not cellulose but mucoproteic.

There have been more interesting studies done with spirulina and pigs. When 5-10% of pig's feed was spirulina a variety of things happened. The reproductive system in males was activated; the number of piglets in each litter increased; birth was easier; and the perinatal mortality was lower. Spirulina has equally good effects on fish. The production of eggs is increased in fish such as trout, salmon and sturgeon, and sexual maturity advanced. And, adding spirulina to the feed of snails resulted in better snails, a lower mortality and stronger shells.

Humans might do well to follow these examples. Already, sportsmen and women have realized that spirulina is particularly useful for vegetarians because it contains a lot of zinc and vitamin B_{12} at the same time. And spirulina has had some results with badly nourished adults and children who were treated at the Bichat

Hospital in Paris, which is in a poor area. So spirulina might well be a food of the future.

Brewer's Yeast

Yeast is a by-product of the beer industry. It is a plant composed of a single cell, about the same size as a blood cell. The American nutritionist Adelle Davis claimed that brewer's yeast could correct most of the dietary problems worldwide just on its own. Brewer's yeast contains an important amount of protein (35% to 50%) and almost all the B vitamins. Also, some kinds of brewer's yeast contain selenium in an organic form which makes it easy to digest. Brewer's yeast contains 7.8mg plus of zinc per 100g. Baker's yeast, which is different, provides 8.0mg zinc in the dried form.

Spirulina and yeast are at the imprecise frontier which separates a diet rich in zinc from the use of supplements.

The Way Ahead for Zinc

The topic of zinc in health is in full flight. It is still a new topic, and what we know at the moment is probably only the tip of the iceberg. Despite this, we know enough to be able to earmark the most promising areas of research for the future.

From the hundreds of medical papers about zinc, certain general rules emerge. It seems that when animals are exposed to a severe zinc deficiency, some organs are affected while others remain completely unaffected. The most vulnerable tissues are those which proliferate most rapidly. This points to future research probably being most fruitful in relation to zinc and skin, the process of growth, reproduction, and the immune system as a whole.

Interestingly, an organ may be very rich in zinc, but unaffected by a shortage of zinc. This seems to be the case with the retina, which is extremely rich in zinc but whose functions of sight are not usually affected by a lack of it. (Although this can happen when a particular anti-tuberculosis drug is used, ethambutamol, which transports zinc away from the retina and affects the sight.)

Zinc has had a fair bit of publicity to do with fertility, preconception, and foetal malformations. But in fact we still have a great deal to learn about intra-uterine growth, preconception and the risks of malformation in the foetus when there is a low level of zinc in the mother. The effects of zinc supplements on human fertility have only been reported anecdotally, likewise with sex therapy. Hardly anything is known either about the role of zinc on the physiological process of childbirth.

Future research will also prove whether or not zinc might protect the male genital organs against the most common degenerative conditions, especially enlarged prostate. Remember that the ancient Chinese used zinc exactly for that purpose. If the ancient Chinese turn out to have been right all along, Western doctors will have made an extremely long detour, via the subtle functions of the metallo-enzymes, to rediscover what others had found out thousands of years ago.

Research in Essential Fatty Acids

Zinc has played a supporting role in many studies to do with essential fatty acids, as zinc is an important catalyst of the metabolic pathway of the unsaturated fatty acids and the synthesis of prostaglandins. Many of these research studies have concentrated on evening primrose oil, as it is a very rich source of GLA (gammalinolenic acid).

In practically every condition for which evening primrose oil has proved successful, zinc (plus vitamin B_6, vitamin C, magnesium and nicotinic acid) needs to be taken too.*

Certainly, taking evening primrose oil, zinc, and the other nutrients seems to be a more sensible first option than the usual drugs prescribed by doctors for these conditions. Other conditions for which this regime has proved useful, but which have not been discussed in detail in this book, are some forms of obesity, heart disease and vascular disorders, and alcoholism.

Zinc and Public Health

It is well known that the greatest stride forward in improving the general health of populations was to do with the introduction of

* For the full range of conditions read Evening Primrose Oil by Judy Graham, published by Thorsons.

safe drinking water, and efficient plumbing to take away effluent. What has to be done now to make that stride complete is make sure the pipes which carry that water are safe. The way forward is to question the use of copper pipes, since we now know that some copper gets into the drinking water, and we need more zinc as a result.

Knowing more about zinc might also prompt some public health organizations to question some agricultural practices, such as the wide use of chemical fertilizers. Every living creature is affected by the impoverishment of soils. Public health and ecology cannot be disassociated.

Wider Issues

There are some common medical practices which actually increase a person's need for zinc in a pathological way. These need to be called into question, particularly those things done in the name of obstetrics and neonatology. Mother and baby are commonly separated during periods of great vulnerability. These separations are factors in depression, both in the short and long term. They create hormonal imbalances which are big consumers of zinc and its co-factors.

The main emphasis of this book has been the variable needs for zinc, and why, ironically, modern man needs more zinc than ever before at the very time when his diet is better than it was. The many reasons why we do need more zinc in our modern society challenges both the way we live today, and modern medicine.

We are at a time when the role of practising medicine appears less important than it was commonly thought to be in the fluctuating health of populations. We are also at a time when conventional medical attitudes are beginning to collapse; attitudes whereby doctors treat symptoms, without understanding that a symptom is a sign that the body is trying to heal itself.

Medicine which treats hypertension with hypotensive drugs; which treats rheumatism with anti-inflammatory drugs, fever by anti-pyretics and behavioural problems with neuroleptic drugs is condemned. Most of these methods first inhibit a physiological function. It is medicine of the past. The kind of medicine which depresses the capacity of adaptation of a patient to cure the disease has what must be considered to be a very negative balance sheet.

At the same time, however, a new kind of medicine is emerging, the 'Nouvelle Medicine' we have suggested, where the priorities are different. Its first aim is to find out the real needs of individuals and populations, and to help and encourage failing physiological processes.

But one has to ask: Why are there so many failing physiological processes in our society? This is the fundamental question. Modern science is understanding better and better how some emotional situations can disturb our systems of adaptation from the beginning of life, and so modify our dietary needs. From lack of love . . . to lack of zinc . . .

References

Chapter 1

Allen, J. I., Korchik, W., Kay, N.E., 'Zinc and T lymphocyte function in hemodialysis patients' Am. J. Clin. Nutr. 36: 410-415 (1982).

Antoniou, L. D., Shalhoub, R. J., Schechter, G. P., 'The effects of zinc on cellular immunity in chronic uremia' Am. J. Clin. Nutr. 34: 1912-1917 (1981).

Beach, R. S., Gershwin, M. E., Makishina, R. K., 'Impaired immunologic ontogeny in post natal zinc deficiency' J. Nutr. 110: 805-815.

Beach, R. S., Gershwin, M. E., Hurley, L. S., 'Altered thymic structure and mitogen responsiveness in post-natally zinc-deficient mice' Dev. Comp. Immunol. 3: 725-738 (1979).

Bjorksten, B., Bach, O., Gustavson, K. H., 'Zinc and immune function in Down's syndrome' Acta paediatr. Scand. 69: 183-187 (1980).

Briggs, W. A., Pedersen, M. M., Mafafan, S. K., 'Lymphocyte and granulocyte function in zinc-treated and zinc deficient hemodialysis patients' Kidney Int. 21: 827-832.

Chvapi, M., Stankova, L., Zukosski, C., 'Inhibition of some functions of polymorphonuclear leucocytes by in vitro zinc' J. Lab. Clin. Med. 89: 135-146 (1977).

Cunnane, S. C., Horrobin, D. F., Manku, M. S., 'Essential fatty acids of zinc deficient rats' Proc. Soc. Exp. Biol. Med. 177: 441-6 (1984).

Czerwinski, A. W., Clark, M. L., Serafetinides, E. A., Perrier, C., Huber,

W., 'Safety of zinc sulphate in geriatric patients' *Clinical Pharmacology and Therapeutics* 15: 436-441 (1974).

Duchateau, J., Delespesse, G., Vereecke, P., 'Influence of oral zinc supplementation on the lymphocyte response to mitogens of normal subjects' A*m. J. Clin. Nutr.* 34: 88-93.

Duchateau, J., Delespesse, G., Vrijeus, R., Collet, H., 'Beneficial effects of oral zinc supplementation on the immune response of old people' A*m. J. Med.* 70: 1001-1004 (1981).

Fenton, M. R., Burke, J. P., Miller, M. L., 'The effects of a zinc deficient diet on the enzymetic activity of rat neutrophils' *Nutr. Reports Int.* 22: 323-328 (1980).

Fraker, P. J., Zwickl, C. M., Luecke, R. W., 'Delayed type hypersensitivity in zinc deficient adult mice' *Proc. Soc. Expl. Biol. Med.* 167: 333-337 (1981).

Fraker, P. S., 'Zinc deficiency: a common immunodeficiency state' *Surv. Immunol. Res.* 2: 155-63 (1983).

Cross, R. L., Osdin, N., Fong, L., 'Depressed immunological function in zinc deprived rats as measured by mitogen response of spleen, thymus and peripheral blood' A*m. J. Clin. Nutr.* 32: 1260-1265 (1979).

Hildebrandt, K. M., Luecke, R. W., Fraker, P. J., 'Effects of maternal dietary zinc on growth and mitogenic responsiveness in suckling mice' *J. Nutr.* 112: 1921-1928 (1982).

Horrobin, D. F. et al., 'The nutritional regulation of T lymphocyte function' *Medical Hypotheses* 5: 969-985 (1979).

Jama 'Taste and smell deviations: importance of zinc' Editorial 24 June, vol. 228 no. 13 (1974).

Mankad, V. N., Ronnlund, R. D., Suskind, R. M., 'Increased immune function in sickle cell disease patients after zinc therapy' *Pediatr. Res.* 17: 237 A (1983).

May, J. M., Cortoreggi, C., 'The mechanism of the insulin-like effects of ionic zinc' *J. Biol. Chem.* 257: 4362-4368 (1982).

Muerheke, R. C., 'The fingernails in hypoalbuminuria: a new physical sign' *Br. Med. J.* 195: 1327-1328 (1956).

O'Dell, B. L., Reynolds, G., Reeves, P. G., 'Analogous effects of zinc deficiency and aspirin toxicity in pregnant rats' *J. Nutr.* 107: 1222-8 (1977).

Prasad, A. S., 'Deficiency of zinc in man and its toxicity' pp 1-20 *Trace Elements in Human Health and Disease* (Prasad and Oberleas eds.) (Academic Press, London 1976).

Sandstead, H. H., Prasad, A. S., Schubert, A. R., 'Human zinc deficiency, endocrine manifestations and response to treatment' *Am. J. Clin. Nutr.* 20: 422-442 (1967).

Scott, G., Ward, R., Wright, D., Robinson, J., Ownubalili, J., Ganci, C., 'Effects of cloned interferon alpha 2 in normal volunteers: febrile reactions and changes in circulating corticosteroids and trace metals' *Antimicrob. Agents Chemother.* 23: 589-592 (1983).

Zanaonico, P., Fernandes, G., Good, R. A., 'The differential sensitivity of T cells and B cells mitogenesis to in vitro zinc deficiency cell' *Immunol.* 60: 203-211 (1981).

Zukoski, C. F., Chvapil, M., Carlson, E., 'Functional immobilization of peritoneal macrophages by zinc' *J. Resiculoendothel. Soc.* 16: 6a (1974).

Zwickel, C. M., Fraker, P. S., 'Restoration of the antibody mediated response of zinc caloric deficient neonatal mice' *Immunol. Commun.* 9: 611-626 (1980).

Chapter 2

Bach, J. F., 'The multifaceted zinc dependency of the immune system' *Immunology To-day* 2: 225-227 (1981).

Chandra, R. K., Dayton, D. H., 'Trace element regulating immunity and infection' *Nutr. Res.* 2: 155-63 (1982).

Chapter 3

Mervyn, L., *The Dictionary of Minerals* (Thorsons, 1985).

Ministry of Agriculture Fisheries and Food, 'Survey of copper and zinc in food' (Food surveillance paper no 5) H M Stationery Office, (1981).

Riordan, J. F., 'Biochemistry of zinc' *Med. Clin. North-Am.* 60: 661 (1976).

Solomons, N. W., 'Biological availability of zinc in humans' *Am. J. Clin. Nutr.* 35: 1048 (1975).

Solomons, N. W., Pineda, O., Viteri, F., Sandstead, H. H., 'Studies on the bioavailability of zinc in humans; mechanism of the intestinal interaction of nonhaem. iron and zinc' *J. Nutr.* 113: 337-49 (1983).

Swanson, C. A., Turnlund, J. R., King, J. C., 'Effect of dietary zinc sources and pregnancy on zinc utilization in adult women fed controlled diets' *J. Nutr.* 113: 2557-2567 (1983).

Chapter 4

Aggett, P. J., Harries, J. T., 'Current status of zinc in health and disease state' *Arch. Dis. Child.* 54: 909-17 (1979).

Antonson, D. L., Van der Hoof, J. A., 'Effect of chronic ethanol ingestion on zinc absorption in rat small intestine' *Dig. Dis. Sci.* 28: 604-08 (1983).

Arakawa, T., Tamura, T., Igarashi, H., Suzuki, H., Sandstead, H., 'Zinc deficiency in two infants during total parenteral alimentation for diarrhoea' *Am. J. Clin. Nutr.* 29: 197 (1976).

Baer, M. T., King, J. C., 'Tissue zinc levels and zinc excretion during experimental zinc depletion in young men' *Am. J. Clin. Nutr.* 39: 556-570 (1984).

Briggs, M. H., Austin, J., Briggs, M., 'Effects of steroid pharmaceuticals on plasma zinc' *Nature* 232-480 (1971).

Craig, W. J., Balbach, L., Harris, S., Vyhmeister, N., 'Plasma zinc and copper levels of infants fed different milk formulas' *J. Am. Coll. Nutr.* 3: 183-6 (1984).

Evans, G. W., Johnson, P. E., 'Characterization and quantitation of a zinc binding ligand in human milk' *Pediatr. Res.* 14: 876-80 (1980).

Fell, G. S., Fleck, A., Cuthertson, D. P., 'Urinary zinc levels as indication of muscle catabolism' *Lancet* 1: 280-282 (1973).

Greger, J. L., Snedeker, S. M., 'Effect of dietary protein and phosphorus levels on the utilization of zinc, copper and manganese by adult males' *J. Nutr.* 110: 2243-2253 (1980).

Halsted, J. A., Smith, Jr., Irvin, M. I., 'A conspectus of research on zinc requirements of man' *J. Nutr.* 104: 345 (1974).

Helwig, H. L., Heffer, E. M., Thulen, W. C., 'Urinary and serum zinc levels in chronic alcoholism' *Am. J. Clin. Pathol* 45: 156-59 (1966).

Jones, R. B., Keeling, P. W. N., Hilton, P. J., Thompson, R. P. H., 'The relationship between leucocyte and muscle zinc in health and disease' *Clin. Sci.* 60: 237-239 (1981).

Kay, R. G. G., Tasman-Jones, C., 'Acute zinc deficiency in man during intravenous alimentation' *Aust. New Zealand J. Surg.* 45: 325 (1975).

Klevay, L. M., 'Hair as a biopsy material. Assessment of zinc nutriture' *Am. J. Clin. Nutr.* 23: 284 (1970).

Lonnerdal, B., Keen, C., Hurley, L. S., 'Zinc binding ligands and complexes in zinc metabolism' *Adv. Nutr. Res.* 6: 139-67 (1984).

MacClain, C. J., Su, L. C., 'Zinc deficiency in the alcoholic: a review' *Alcoholism Clin. Res.* 7: 5-10 (1983).

Murphy, B. F., Gray, O. P., Rendall, J. R., Hann, S., 'Zinc deficiency: a problem with preterm breast milk' *Early Human Det.* 10: 303-7 (1985).

Principi, N., Giuntasa, A., Gervasoni, A., 'The role of zinc in total parenteral nutrition' *Acta. Paediatr. Scand.* 68: 129 (1979).

Recommended Dietary Allowances (8th ed.) National Academy of Sciences, Washington D C, (1974).

Seal, C. J., Heaton, F. W., 'Chemical factors affecting the intestinal absorption of zinc in vitro and in vivo'. *Br. J. Nutr.* 50: 317-24 (1983).

Southon, S., Gee, J. M., Johnson, I. T., 'Intestinal uptake of galactose in rats recovering from experimental zinc deficiency' *Proc. Nut. Soc.* 43: 90 A (1983).

Southon, S., Gee, J. M., Johnson, I. T., 'Hexode transport and mucosal morphology in the small intestine of the zinc deficient rat' *B. J. Nutr.* 52: 371-80 (1984).

Turnlund, J. R., King, J. C., Keyes, W. R., Gong, B., Michel, M. C., 'A stable isotope study of zinc absorption in young men: effects of phytate and alpha-cellulose' *Am. J. Clin. Nutr.* 40: 1071-1077 (1984).

Underwood, E. J., 'Trace elements in human and animal nutrition (4th ed.) (Academic Press, London 1977).

Chapter 5

Brummerstead, Flagstad, Bass, 'The effect of zinc on calves with hereditary thymus hypoplasia' *Acta. Pathol. Microbiol. Scand.* 79: 686-687 (1971).

Cavdar, A. O., Arcasoy, A., Cin, S., Babacan, E., Gozdasoglu, S., 'Geophagia in Turkey: Iron and zinc deficiency, iron and zinc absorption studies and response to treatment with zinc in geophagia cases' *Prog. Clin. Biol. Res.* 129: 71-97 (1983).

Dahmer, E. J., Grummer, R. H., Hoekstra, W. G., 'Effects of histidine on zinc deficiency in baby pigs' *J. Animal Sci.* 26: 1475 (1967).

Danbolt, N., Closs, K., 'Akrodermatitis enteropathica' *Acta. Derm. Venerol.* 23 (1943).

Dillaha, C. J., Lorinez, A., Aavik, O. R., 'Acrodermatitis enteropathica: review of the literature and report of a case successfully treated with diodoquin' *Jama* 152: 509-512 (1953).

Hambidge, M. K., Neldur, K. H., Wabravens, P. A., 'Acrodermatitis enteropathica and congenital malformations' *Lancet* 1: 577 (1975).

Kelly, R., Davidson, G. P., Kownley, R. R. W., Campbell, P. E., 'Reversible intestinal mucosal abnormalities in acrodermatitis enteropathica' *Arch. Dis. Child.* 51-219 (1976).

Kenneth, H., Neldur, M. D., Hambidge, K. M., 'Zinc therapy of acrodermatitis enteropathica' *The New England Journal of Medicine*, 24 April 1975, pp 879-882.

Michaelson, G., 'Zinc therapy in acrodermatitis enteropathica' *Acta. Derm. Venerol.* (Stockh.) 54: 377-381 (1974).

Moynahan, E. J., 'Acrodermatitis enteropathica' *Lancet* 2: 399-400 (1974). A lethal inherited human zinc deficiency disorder.

Neldur, Hambidge, 'Zinc therapy of acrodermatitis enteropathica' *New Engl. J. Med.* 292: 879-82 (1975).

Prasad, A. S., 'Metabolism of zinc and its deficiency in human subjects' in Prasad, A. S., (ed.): *Zinc Metabolism* p. 302. (Charles C. Thomas, 1966).

Prasad, A. S., Miale, A., Farid, Z., 'Zinc metabolism in normals and patients with the syndrome of iron deficiency anaemia hypogonadism, and dwarfism' *J. Lab. Clin. Med.* 61: 537-549 (1963).

Weismann, K., Flagstad, T., 'Hereditary zinc deficiency (adema disease) in cattle: an animal parallel to acrodermatitis enteropathica' *Acta. Dermato. Venerol.* 56: 151 (1976).

Chapter 6

Apgar, J., 'Effect of zinc deprivation from day 12, 15 or 18 of gestation on parturition in the rat' *J. Nutrition* 102: 343-347 (1972).

Apgar, J., 'Effect of zinc repletion late in gestation on parturition in the zinc deficient rat' *Journal of Nutrition* 103: July 1973.

'Aspirin and preeclampsia' Editorial, *Lancet* 4 January 1986.

Baumslag, N., Yeager, D., Levin, L., Petering, H. G., 'Trace metal content of maternal and neonatal hair, zinc, copper, iron and lead. *Arch. Environ. Health* 29: 186-191 (1974).

Beaufils, M., Uzan, S., Dousimoni, R., Colan, J. C., 'Prevention of preeclampsia by early antiplatelet therapy' *Lancet* 840-42 (1985).

Brewer, T., 'Iatrogenic starvation in human pregnancy' *Medikon International* (Ghent, Belgium) No 4. pp. 14-15. 30 May 1974.

Brewer, T., *Metabolic Toxemia of Late Pregnancy: a disease of malnutrition* (Keats, New Canaan, 1982).

Caldwell, D. F., Oberleas, D., Prasad, A., 'Reproductive performance of chronic mildly zinc deficient rats and the effects on behaviour of their offspring' *Nutr. Rept. Intern.* 7: 309 (1973).

Campbell-Brown, M., Ward, R. J., Haines, A. P., 'Zinc and copper in Asian pregnancies: Is there evidence for a nutritional deficiency?' *Br. J. Obstet. Gynaecol.* 92: 875-85 (1985).

Chester, R., Dukes, M., Slatter, S. R., Walpole, A. L., 'Delay of parturition in the rat by anti-inflammatory agents which inhibit the biosynthesis of prostaglandins' *Nature* 240: 37-38 (1972).

Cramdon, A. J., Ishervood, D. M., 'Effect of aspirin on incidence of preeclampsia' *Lancet* p. 1356 (1979).

Dreosti, I. E., Tao, S. H., Hurley, L. S., 'Plasma zinc and leucocyte changes in weaning and pregnant rats during zinc deficiency' *Proc. Soc. Exp. Biol. Med.* 128: 169-174 (1968).

Dura-Trave, T., Ping-Abuli, N., Moureal, I., Villa-Elisaga, I., 'Relation between material plasmatic zinc levels and uterine contractility' *Gynaecol. Obstet. Invest.* 17: 247-251 (1984).

Fievet, P., Tribout, B., Dieval, J., Capio, J. C., Delobel, J., Fournier, A., Papanicolaou, N., Gregoire, N., 'Effects of evening primrose oil on platelet functions during pregnancy in patients with high risk of toxemia.' Result of a preliminary study. Second International

Congress on Essential Fatty Acids, Prostaglandins and Leukotrienes, London, March 1985.

Ghosh, A., Fong, L. Y. Y., Wan, C. W., Liang, S. T., Woo, J. S. K., Wong, V., 'Zinc deficiency is not a cause for abortion, congenital abnormality and small-for-gestational age infant in Chinese women' Br. J. Obst. Gynaecol. 92: 886-91 (1985).

Hurley, L. S., Gowan, J., Swenerton, H., 'Teratogenic effects of short term and transitory zinc deficiency in rats' Teratology 4: 199-204 (1969).

Hurley, L. S., Swenerton, H., 'Congenital malformations resulting from zinc deficiency in rats' Proc. Soc. Expl. Biol. Med. 123: 692 (1966).

Hyten, F. E., Commentary, 'Do pregnant women need zinc supplements?' Br. J. Obstet. Gynaecol. 92: 873-74 (1985).

Jameson, S., 'Effects of zinc deficiency in human reproduction' Acta. Med. Scand. 593: 4 (1976).

Kulhohma, P., Paul, R., Pakarineu, P., Gronroos, M., 'Copper and zinc in preeclampsia' Acta Obstet. Gynaecol. Scand. 63-67, 629, 631 (1984).

Kumor, S., 'Effects of zinc supplementation on rats during pregnancy' Nutr. Rep. Int. 13: 33-36 (1976).

MacKenzie, J. M., Fosmire, G. J., Sandstead, H. H., 'Zinc deficiency during the latter third of pregnancy: effects on fetal rat brain, liver and placenta' J. Nutr. 105: 1466 (1975).

Meadows, N. J., Ruse, W., Smith, M., Keeling, P. W. N., Blozam, D., Day, J., Scopes, J. W., Thorapson, R. P. H., 'Zinc and small babies' Lancet 2: 1135-1137 (1981).

Misconceptions about preconceptional care (editorial) Lancet 1046, 1047 9 Nov 1985.

O'Dell, B., Reynolds, G., Reeves, P. G., 'Analogous effects of zinc deficiency and aspirin toxicity in the pregnant rat' J. Nutr. 107: 1222-8 (1977).

Pinard, A., 'Esquisse des progres realisés en obstetrique pendant le 19eme siecle' Annales de Gynecologie et d'Obstetrique. (December 1900).

Prema, K., 'Predictive value of serum copper and zinc in normal and abnormal pregnancy' Ind. J. Med. Res. 71: 554-560 (1980).

Sandstead, H. H., Strobel, D. A., Logan, G. M., Marks, E. O., Jacob, R. A., 'Zinc deficiency in pregnant rhesus monkeys: effects on behaviour of infants' *Am. J. Clin. Nutr.* 31: 844-49 (1978).

Sheldon, W. L., Apillaga, M. O., Smith, P. A., Lind, T. 'The effects of oral iron supplementation on zinc and magnesium levels during pregnancy' *Br. J. Obst. Gynaecol.* 92: 892-98 (1985).

Simmer, K., Punchard, N. A., Murphy, G., Thompson, R. P., 'Prostaglandin production and zinc depletion in human pregnancy' *Pediatric. Research* vol. 19 no. 7 (1985).

Simmer, K., Thompson, R. P. H., 'Maternal zinc depletion and intrauterine growth retardation' *Clin. Sci.* 68: 385-399 (1985).

Swenerton, H., Shrader, R., Hurley, L. S., 'Zinc deficiency embryos: reduced thymidine incorporation' *Science* 166: 1014 (1969).

Turnlund, J., King, J., Wahbeh, C. J., Ishkanian, Tannous, R. I., 'Zinc status and pregnancy outcome of pregnant Lebanese women' *Nutr. Res.* 3: 309-315 (1983).

Wallenburg, H. C. S., Dekker, G. A., Makovitz, J. W., Rotmans, P., 'Low dose aspirin prevents pregnancy — induced hypertension and preeclampsia in angiotensin-sensitive primigravidae' *Lancet* pp 1-3, 4 January 1986.

Wallenburg, H. C. S., Rotmans, N., 'Enhanced reactivity of the platelet thromboxane pathway in normotensive and hypertensive pregnancies with insufficient fetal growth' *Am. J. Obstet. Gynecol.* 144: 523-28 (1982).

Walsh, S. W., 'Preeclampsia: an imbalance in placental prostacyclin and thromboxane production' *Am. J. Obstet. Gynecol.* 152: 335-40 (1985).

Warkany, J. Petering, H. G., 'Congenital malformations of the central nervous system in rats produced by maternal zinc deficiency' *Teratology* 5: 319-334 (1972).

Chapter 7

Barnes, B., Colquhoon, J., *The Hyperactive Child* (Thorsons, 1984).

Byron, N. A., Timlin, D. M., 'Immune status in atopic eczema: a survey' *British Journal of Dermatology* 100: 491-498 (1979).

Feingold, B. F., *Why Your Child is Hyperactive* (Random House, N. Y., 1975).

Grant, E., *The Bitter Pill* (Elm Tree Books, 1985).

Lancet Editorial, 'Feingold's regime for hyperkinesis' *Lancet* 2: 617-8 (1979).

Swanson, J. M., Kinsbourne, M., 'Food dyes impair performance of hyperactive children in a laboratory learning test' *Science* 207: 1485-7 (1980).

Tiubergen, N. and E., *Autistic Children: New Hope for a Cure* (Allen and Unwin, London 1983).

Chapter 8

Alvares, O. F., Meyer, J., 'Regional differences in parakeratotic response to mild zinc deficiency' *Arch. Derm.* 98: 191-201 (1968).

Barney, G. H., Macapiulac, M. P., Pearson, W. N., Darby, W. J., 'Parakeratosis of the tongue — a human histopathologic lesion in the zinc deficient squirrel monkey' *J. Nutr.* 93: 511 (1967).

Brody, 'Topical treatment of recurrent herpes simplex and post herpetic erythema multiform with low concentrations of zinc sulphate solution' *Br. J. Dermatol.* 104: 191-194 (1981).

Hoekstra, W. G., 'The relationship of parakeratosis, supplemental calcium and zinc to the zinc content of certain body components of swine' *J. Animal Sci.* 15: 752-764 (1956).

Michaelson, G., 'Effects of oral zinc and vitamin A in acne' *Jama: Archives of Dermatology* 113: 3-36 (1977).

Pories, W. J., Henzel, J. H., Rob, C. G., Strain, W. H., 'Promotion of wound healing in man with zinc sulphate given by mouth' *Lancet* 1: 121-124.

Reaven, E. P., Cox, A. J., 'Binding of zinc by the transitional layer of the epidermis' *J. Invest. Derm.* 39: 133-137 (1962).

Richard, B. F., 'Facial eczema: zinc responsiveness in dairy cattle' *New Zealand Veterinary Journal* vol. 23 pp. 41-3 (1975).

Turcker, H. F., Salmon, W. D., 'Parakeratosis or zinc deficiency disease in the pig' *Proc. Soc. Exp. Biol. Med.* 88: 613-616 (1955).

Voorhees, J. J., Chakrabarti, S. G., Botero, F., Miedler, L., Harrell, E. R., 'Zinc therapy and distribution in psoriasis' *Arch. Derm.* vol. 100 (1969).

Wahaba, A., 'Topical application of zinc solution: a new treatment for herpes simplex infections of the skin' *Acta. Derm. Venerol.* 60: 175-177 (1980).

Chapter 9

Bogomolva, G. G., Karluskil, V. M., 'Indices of zinc metabolism in leukemias' *Vrach. Delo.* 12: 57-61 (1977).

Butterworth, B. E., Grunert, R. R., Korant, B. D., Louberg-Holm, K., Yin, F. H., 'Replication of rhinoviruses' *Arch. Virol.* 51: 169-189.

Butterworth, B. E., Korant, B. D., 'Characterization of the large picornoviral polypeptides produced in the presence of zinc ion' *J. Virol.* 14: 282-291.

Eby, G. A., Davis, D. R., Halcomb, W. W., 'Reduction in duration of common colds by zinc gluconate lozenges in a double-blind study' *Antimicrobiol. Agents and Chemotherapy.* vol. 25 no. 1 pp. 20-24, Jan 1984.

Korant, B. D., Butterworth, B. E., 'Inhibition by zinc of rhinovirus protein cleavage: interaction of zinc with capsid polypeptides' *J. Virol.* 18: 298-306 (1976).

Korant, B. D., Kaner, J. C., Butterworth, B. E., 'Zinc ions inhibit replication of rhinoviruses' *Nature* 248: 588-590 (1974).

Chapter 10

Adam, E., Rawls, W. E., Melnik, J. L., 'The association of herpes virus 2 infection and cervical cancer' *Prev. Med.* 3 (1974).

Baker, D. A., Thomas, J., 'The effect of prostaglandins E2 on the initial immune response to herpes simplex virus infection' *Am. J. Obst. Gynecol.* 151: 586-590 (1985).

Becker, W. B., Kipps, A., McKenzie, D., 'Disseminated herpes simplex virus infection: Its pathogenesis based on virological and pathological studies in 33 cases' *Am. J. Dis. Child* 115: 1-8 (1968).

Binkin, N. J., Koplan, J. P., Cates, W., Jr., 'Preventing neonatal herpes: the value of viral cultures in pregnant women with recurrent genital herpes' *Jama.* 251: 2816-21 (1984).

Brody, I., 'Topical treatment of recurrent herpes simplex and post-herpetic erythema multiforme with low concentrations of zinc sulphate solution' Br. J. Dermatol. 104: 191-194 (1981).

Fahim, M. S., Browner, T. A., and Hall, D. G., 'New treatment for herpes simplex virus type 2 (ultrasound and zinc, urea and tannic acid ointment). Part II: Female patients' J. Med. (Westbury) 11: 143-167 (1980).

Fridlender, B., Chejanovsky, N., and Becker, Y., 'Selective inhibitions of herpes simplex virus type 1 D N A polymerase by zinc ions' Virology 84: 551-554.

Frazier, J. P., Kohl, S., Pickering, L. K. et al 'The effect of route of delivery on neonatal natural killer cytotoxicity and antibody-dependant cellular cytotoxicity to herpes simplex virus-infected cell' Pediatr. Res. 558-560 (1982).

Gordon, Y. J., Asher, Y., Becker, Y., 'Irreversible inhibition of herpes simplex virus replication in B C S — 1 cells by zinc irons' Antimicrobiol Agents and chemotherapy 8: 377 (1975).

Gupta, P., and Rapp, F., 'Effect of zinc ions on synthesis of herpes simplex virus type 2 — induced polypeptides' Proc. Soc. Biol. Med. 152: 455-458 (1976).

Hill, T. S., Field, H. J., Blyth, W. A., 'Acute and recurrent infection with herpes simplex virus in the mouse: a model for studying latency and recurrent disease' J. Gen. Virol. 28: 341 (1975).

Kohl, S., 'Defective infant antiviral cytotoxicity to herpes simplex virus-infected cells' J. Pediatr. 102: 885-888 (1983).

Nahmias, A. J., Dowdle, W. R., Josey, W. E., et al 'Newborn infection with herpes virus hominis types 1 and 2' J. Pediatr. 75: 1194-1203 (1969).

Shlornal, J., Asher, Y., Gordon, Y. J., Olshervsky, U., Becker, Y., 'Effect of zinc ions on the synthesis of herpes simplex virus D N A in infected B C C 1 cells' Virology 66: 330 (1975).

Tennican, P. O., cited Marks, R. G., New hope in herpes genitalis current prescribing. 3: 27 (1979).

Wahba, A., 'Topical application of zinc solutions: a new treatment for herpes simplex infections of the skin?' Acta. Derm. Venereol. 60: 175-177 (1980).

Warford, A. L., Levy, R. A., Rekrut, K. A., Steinberg, E., 'Herpes simplex virus testing of an obstetric population with an antigen enzyme-linked immunosorbent assay' *American Journal of Obstetrics and Gynecology* 154: 21-28 (1986).

Chapter 11

Akar, N., 'Anorexia and zinc' *Lancet* p. 874 (1984).

Amstrong, Esther C. A., Lacey, J. H., Crisp, A. H., Bryant, T. N., 'An investigation of the immune response of patients suffering from anorexia nervosa' *Postgrad. Med. J.* 54: 395-9 (1978).

Bakan, R., 'Anorexia and zinc' *Lancet* p. 874 (13 Oct 1984).

Bakan, R., 'The role of zinc in anorexia nervosa: aetiology and treatment' *Med. Hypoth.* 5: 731-36 (1979).

Bryce-Smith, D., 'Case of anorexia nervosa responding to zinc sulphate' *Lancet* p. 350 (11 Aug 1984).

Bryce-Smith, D., Simpson, R. I. D., 'Anorexia, depression and zinc deficiency' *Lancet* p. 1162 (17 Nov 1984).

Chesters, J. K., Quarterman, J., 'Effects of zinc deficiency on food intake and feeding patterns of rats' *Brit. J. Nutr.* 24: 1061 (1970).

Dinsmore, W. W., Alderdice, J. T., MacMasher, Dorothy, Adams, C. E. A., Love, A. H. G., 'Zinc absorption in anorexia nervosa' *Lancet* pp. 1041-1042 (4 May 1985).

Garfinkel, P. E., Garner, D. M., *Anorexia Nervosa*, (Brummer/Mazel, New York 1982).

Golla, J. A., Larson, L. A., Anderson, C. F., Lucas, A. R., Wilson, W. R., Tomassi, T. B., 'An immunological assessment of patients with anorexia nervosa' *Am. J. Clin. Nutr.* 34: 2756-62 (1981).

Horrobin, D. F., Cunnane, S. C., 'Interactions between zinc, essential fatty acids and prostaglandins. Relevance to acrodermatitis enteropathica, total parenteral nutrition, the glucagonoma syndrome, diabetes, anorexia nervosa and sickle cell anemia' *Med. Hypoth.* 6: 277-96 (1980).

Lupton, M., Simon, L., Barry, V., Klawans, H. L., 'Biological aspects of anorexia nervosa' *Life Sci.* 18: 1341 (1976).

Pertschuk, M. J., Crosby, L. O., Barot, L., Muller, J. L.,

'Immunocompetency in anorexia nervosa' *Am. J. Clin. Nutr.* 35: 968-72 (1982).

Chapter 12

Beck, A., Sethi, B., Tuthill, R., 'Childhood bereavement and adult depression' *Archives of General Psychiatry* 9: 295-302 (1963).

Brown, F., 'Depression and childhood bereavement' *Journal of Mental Sciences* 107: 755-777.

Kronfol, Ziad, House, J. D., 'Depression, cortisol and immune function' *Lancet* pp. 1026-1027 (5 May 1984).

Chapter 13

Rheumatism

Benhamon, C. L., Brandeley, M., 'Influence de la grossesse et de l'état hormonal sur la polyarthrite rhumatoide' *Presse Medicale* no. 36, 2223-2224 (15 Oct 1983).

Horrobin, D. F., 'The regulation of prostaglandin biosynthesis: Negative feedback mechanisms and the selective control of formation of 1 and 2 series prostaglandins: relevance to inflammation and immunity' *Medical Hypotheses* 6: 687-799 (1980).

Simkin, P. A., 'Oral zinc sulphate in rheumatoid arthritis' *Lancet* pp. 539-542 (1976).

Zurier, R. B., Quagliata, F., 'Effect of prostaglandins E1 on adjuvant arthritis' *Nature* 234: 304-305 (1971).

Schizophrenia

Abdulla, Y. H., Hamadah, K., 'Effect of A D P on P G E formation in blood platelets from patients with depression, mania, schizophrenia' *B. J. Psychiatry* 127: 591-5 (1975).

Goldstein, A. L., Rossio, J., Koliaskina, G. L., Emory, L. E., Overall, J. B., Thurman, G. B., Hatchur, J., 'Immunological components in schizophrenia. Perspectives in schizophrenia research' pp. 249-267 (Raven Press, New York, 1980).

Horrobin, D. F., 'Schizophrenia as a prostaglandin deficiency disease' *Lancet* 1: 936-937 (1977).

Horrobin, D. F., 'Schizophrenia: reconciliation of the dopamine prostaglandin and opioid concepts: role of the pineal' *Lancet* 1: 529-531 (1979).

Pfeiffer, C. C., Iliet, V., 'A study of zinc deficiency and copper excess in the schizophrenic' *Int. Ref. Neurobiol.* suppl. 1. 1972.

Watamebe, M., Funakashi, T., Suzuki, T., Nomura, S., Nakazawa, T., Noguchi, T., Tsukada, Y., 'Antithymic antibodies in schizophrenic sera' *Biological Psychiatry* 17: 699-710 (1982).

Chapter 14

Clement, G., 'Une nouvelle ressource: L'algue spiruline' *Soc. Phycol. de France Bull* no. 23 (1978).

Murphy, J. V., 'Intoxication following ingestion of elemental zinc' *Jama* 212: 2119-2120 (1970).

Nichols, B. W., Wood, B. J., 'The occurrence and biosynthesis of gamma linolenic acid in a blue green algae, spirulina platensis' *Lipids* vol. 3 pp 346-50 (Jan 1968).

Pfeiffer, C. C., Papaioannoce, R., Sobler, A., 'Effect of chronic zinc intoxication on copper levels, blood formation and polyamines' *Orthomol. Psychiatry* 9: 79-89 (1980).

Chapter 15

Averback, P., 'Anencephaly associated with megavitamin therapy' *Can. Med. Assoc. J.* 114: 995 (1976).

Bettger, W. J., O'Dell, B. L., 'A critical physiological role of zinc in the structure and function of biomembranes' *Life Sci.* 28: 1425-1438 (1981).

Fair, W. R., Heston, W., 'Prostate inflammation linked to zinc shortage' *Prevention* p. 113 (June 1977).

Krieger, I., Alpern, B. E., Cunnane, S. C., 'Transient neonatal zinc deficiency' *Am. J. Clin. Nutr.* (1986).

Manku, M. S., Horrobin, D. F., Karmazin, M., Cunnane, S. C., 'Prolactin and zinc effects on rat vascular reactivity: possible relationship to dihomogammalinolenic acid and to prostaglandins synthesis' *Endocrinology* vol. 104 No. 3 (1979).

Moynahan, E. J., 'Zinc deficiency and disturbances of mood and visual behaviour' *Lancet* 1/10, 91 (1976).

Song, M. K., Adham, N. F., Ament, M. E., 'Evidence for a role of prostaglandins in the regulation of intestinal zinc transport' *Nutrition Reports International* (1985).

Index